This Journal Belongs To:

Name ....

Email ....

Telephone ....

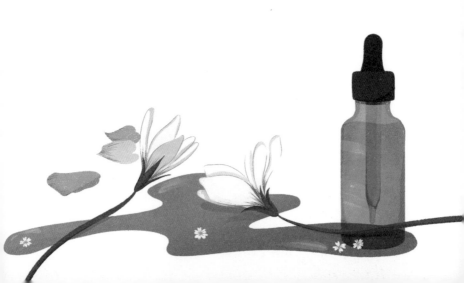

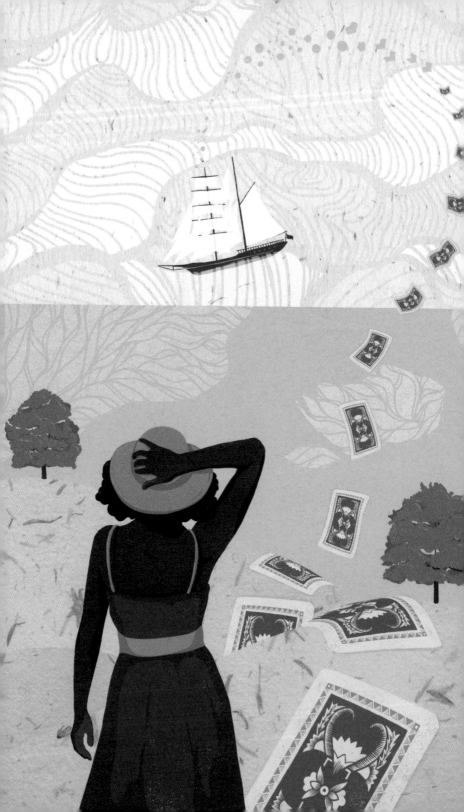

Breathe

Happiness

JOURNAL

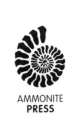

AMMONITE
PRESS

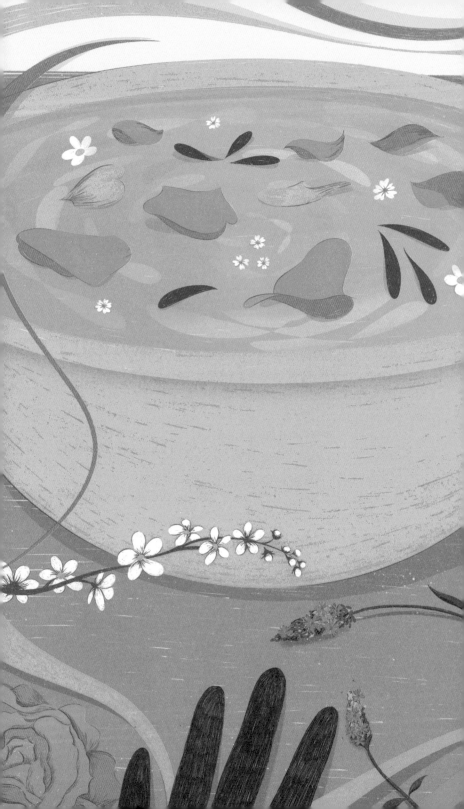

Happiness

Happiness can mean so many things. It can be found in personal achievement, or in letting go of expectations. Some might discover it in noticing the small pleasures of everyday, others by remembering they're part of something bigger than themselves.

There are as many recipes for happiness as there are people hoping for a taste of it, but there are certain key ingredients that appear time and again. This journal explores some of these, from connecting with others, engaging the senses and immersion in the natural world to self-compassion, awareness of life's transience and practising gratitude. It includes examples of how to tap into your creativity, suggestions for how to engage more deeply with the world and space to examine your own ideas about what might bring you joy. Use it to kickstart your exploration of what happiness means.

Breathe

breathemagazine.com

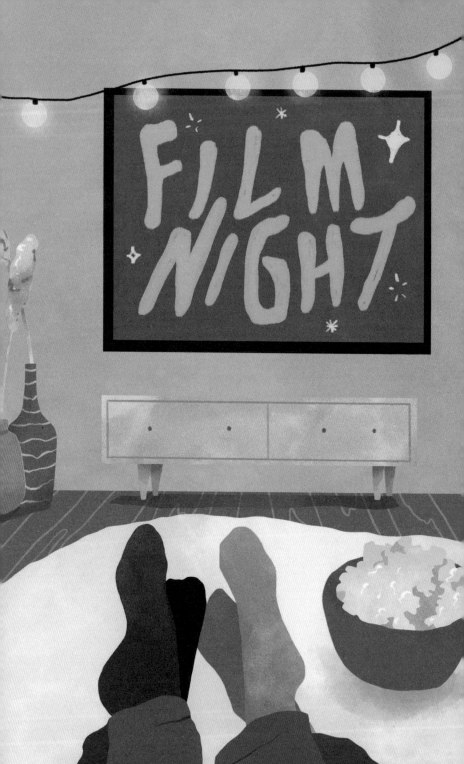

Contents

What is happiness?

It's a very human thing to want to be happy, but few people know exactly what they mean when they say it, much less how to find this state of being or hold on to it

Search for the word 'happiness' on the internet and you'll find any number of websites telling you how to find it. Looking for happiness is, according to Aristotle, 'the meaning and the purpose of life, the whole aim and end of human existence.' It's the most human of goals, one that's even listed in the United States Declaration of Independence, but judging by the number of self-help sites out there, it's also one that many people are struggling to attain.

So, what is it, this mysterious state of being? Is it in your genes or does it come from your environment? And what are you supposed to do to live a happy life?

Understanding happiness

Ask people to define happiness and, depending on their past experiences, the culture that has shaped them, their environment and the time they're living in, they'll give you different answers. In other words, what makes you happy won't necessarily provoke the same feeling in another person.

Because people interpret happiness in different ways, it's difficult to give a definition that's true for everyone. Nevertheless, there are different kinds of happiness depending on different factors, from social (the pleasure of being with family and friends) and vocational (a satisfying job) to physical (good health) and materialistic (basically anything you want to own).

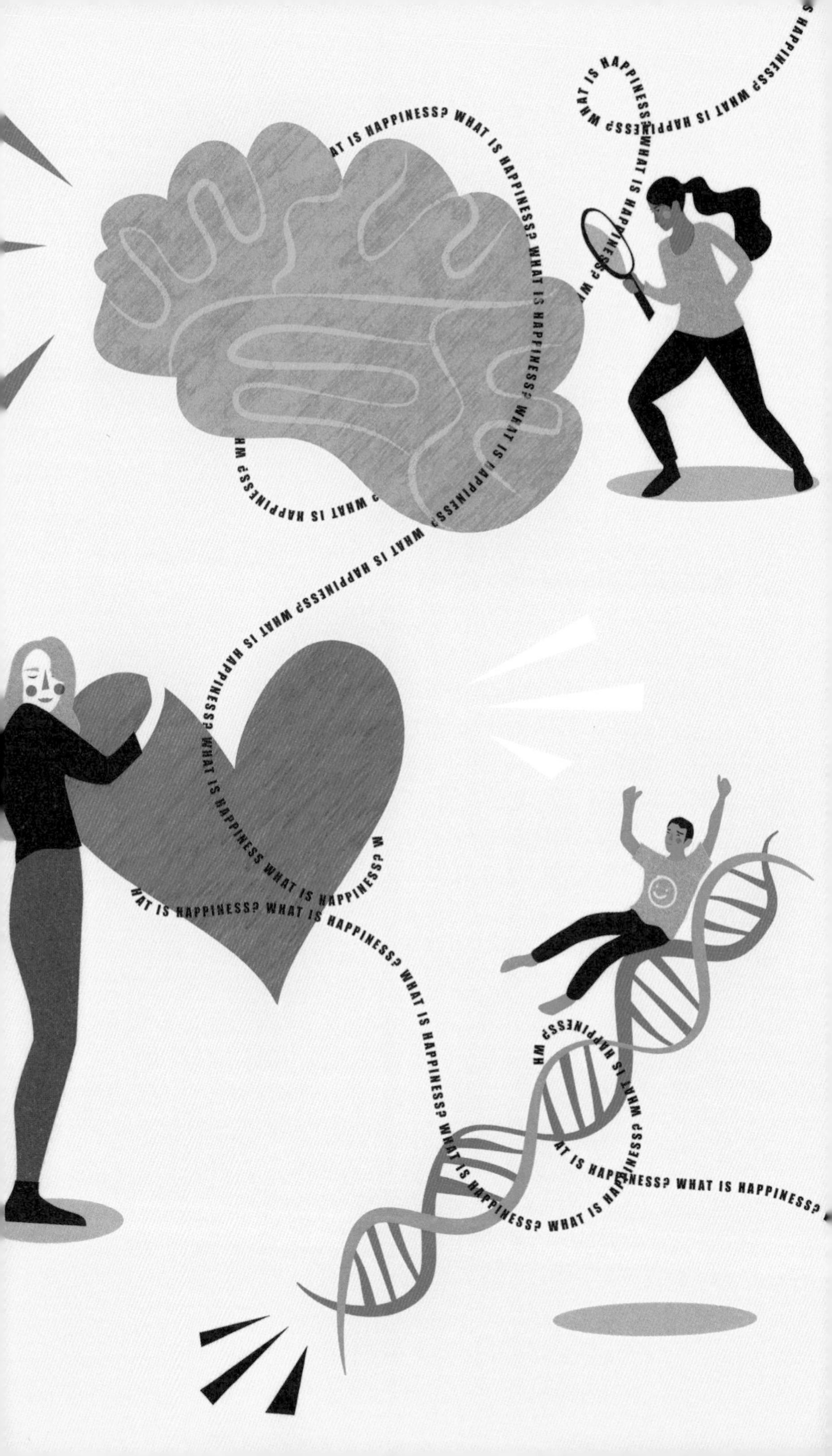
WHAT IS HAPPINESS? WHAT IS HAPPINESS? WHAT IS HAPPINESS? WHAT IS HAPPINESS? WHAT IS HAPPINESS?

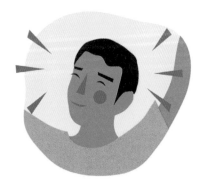

The science of happiness

The heart is often linked to happiness – 'My heart is going to burst' or 'My heart is filled with joy' – yet the real source is not the heart but the brain. Taking a (neuro) scientific approach, it's possible to explore what really happens when you feel contentment, as the brain releases 'happy' chemicals, which affect people in different ways:

- Dopamine plays a role in pleasure and reward behaviour.
- Serotonin acts as a mood stabiliser and prevents depression.
- Endorphins possess morphine-like effects and block pain.
- Oxytocin provides feelings of love and trust.

By understanding how these chemicals originate, you can stimulate your brain to produce more of them, by creating daily experiences that activate them and elevate your level of happiness.

The United Nations now publishes an annual World Happiness Report, reviewing the state of the world's happiness, and suggests governments pay attention to it, as happiness plays an important role in the health and productivity of a nation. And, as advances in neuroscience unlock many of the brain's mysteries, wellbeing has become the topic of an increasing number of scientific studies.

Some of these studies have even looked at whether DNA is a key to happiness. If certain people are prone to depression, are others literally born to be happy? Researchers have recently uncovered a genetic link and concluded that nations with the highest prevalence of a particular DNA code have the highest percentages of happy people.

While it may be impossible to change your DNA, you can influence your environment and the way you respond to it. Science has proved that you can take control and adjust the chemical balance in your brain, to cultivate and sustain positive emotions. People are naturally wired to pay more attention to negative experiences, but they are not doomed, good DNA or not, as it's possible to rewire the brain to be more aware of the positive using simple techniques, such as mindfulness, practising gratitude and physical exercise.

THE SECRET TO HAPPINESS

While the personal nature of happiness makes it difficult to pin down, the dictionary defines it as: A mental or emotional state of wellbeing defined by positive or pleasant emotions, ranging from contentment to intense joy.

In other words, a happy life starts from within. It may be influenced by external circumstances and genetics, but it's mainly dependent on you, your actions and your thoughts. It's a conscious choice and a state of mind that can be cultivated. The more you understand how your brain works, the more you gain the ability to change the way you think – and feel.

A good place to start is by getting to know yourself better. This involves trying to work out what your biggest sources of happiness and unhappiness are, then looking at changes that might impact these.

Do you know what makes you happy? Can you describe it?

....

....

....

....

....

....

....

....

....

....

....

....

How do you feel about your life right now?

....

....

....

....

....

....

Describe times when you feel relaxed and calm

....

....

....

....

....

....

Describe times when you feel worried or anxious

....

....

....

....

....

....

List the times you did something just for fun in the last month

....

....

....

....

....

Reading back over your answers, do they make you feel content and optimistic or are there areas where the negative outweighs the positive? Are there new opportunities you could introduce to enrich your everyday life? Are you looking after yourself? What changes could you make that might improve how you feel?

....

....

....

....

....

....

....

....

....

....

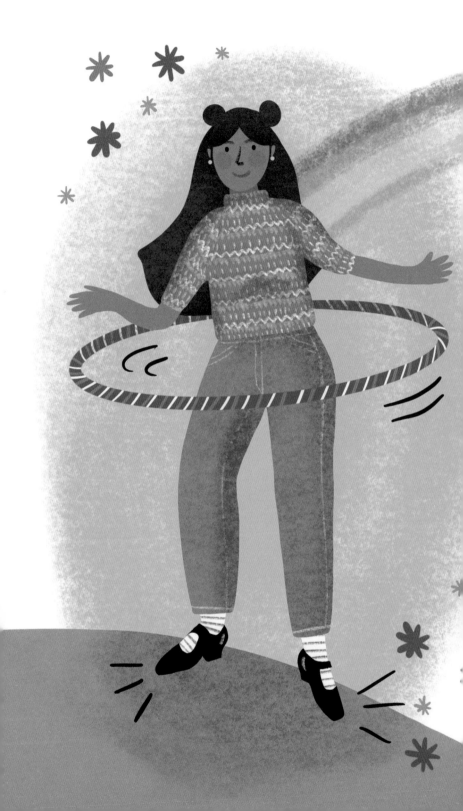

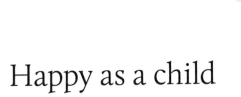

Happy as a child

Whether it's collecting stamps or tap-dancing, revisiting a childhood passion can open up a whole new world of wonder

Watching a child absorbed in a game or simple task, a contented look on their face and an easy relaxation in their body, is a valuable reminder of how much can be learned by revisiting the things that brought you joy as a child. Many people have found that by reconnecting with childhood pleasures, they can, wonderfully, experience the same level of enjoyment from those activities as they did years ago.

A happier mind

Shamash Alidina is a co-founder of the Museum of Happiness in London, as well as a mindfulness trainer, lecturer and author of *Mindfulness for Dummies*. Many of the museum's events recreate fun childhood activities. Shamash explains the reasoning behind this: 'Rediscovering our joys of childhood is a journey back to coming into the moment. Our minds spend around 50 per cent of the time thinking, planning and, most often, worrying. By doing fun activities, you bring your attention from your worries to the present moment. A mind that is more in the present moment is a happier mind.'

It often takes trying out something in a different environment to rediscover a love for a childhood activity. Perhaps taking a sketch pad along to your favourite café for a mindful doodle while enjoying a coffee, or joining in with the hula-hooping masterclass at the local summer fête.

Rachel Hard is a registered psychologist who often encourages clients struggling with mental and emotional challenges, such as stress, anxiety and depression, to reconnect with the activities they enjoyed most as children. 'Adulting is hard,' she says. 'There's something nostalgic about childhood games that really reminds us of those halcyon days – a time with less responsibility and worry. It's not only a way to counteract those [negative] feelings, but also helps us to reconnect with a time when we felt more carefree.'

Keep it fun

There's no need to look for something transformative, and the activity itself doesn't matter, as long as it's something you enjoy. Many childhood interests are absorbing and have elements of creativity and repetition, such as dancing, cross-stitch or playing solitaire. This means not having to think too much about what you're doing – unlike many adult activities that involve huge mental effort. Rachel explains why this can be helpful: 'We can focus on the task at hand and don't need to do a lot of processing or assessment. Our minds can only focus on a finite number of things… so if we distract ourselves with simple and fun activities, we can block out other thoughts or negative thought patterns.'

The fun element helps to manage debilitating patterns such as overthinking and worrying. Shamash explains how this works: 'The wandering mind activates a part of a network of the brain called the default mode network. This can link up to your fear centre – your amygdala – creating cycles of worry and anxiety. Through being more childlike and playful or doing a calming present-moment activity, you shift to a more present, moment-focused network in your brain, get less caught up in negative cycles of rumination and build greater emotional resilience.'

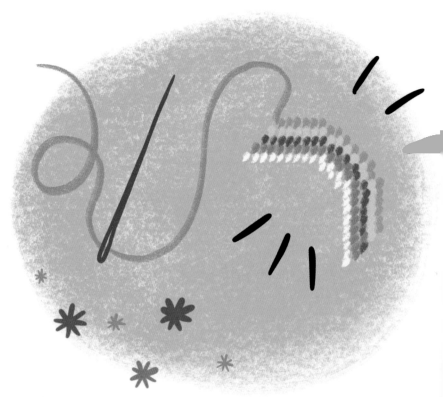

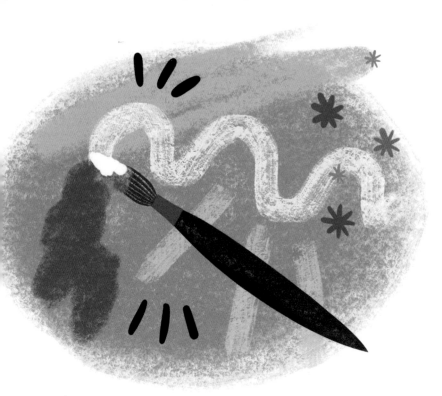

Focus on the process

Professional artist Rebecca Steels-Hargreaves, from York, rediscovered her childhood passion for painting as something to help her through a time of major life changes. 'As a child I would draw and paint for hours... I loved the escape,' she says. 'I went on to study graphic design, yet painting had been my childhood passion, though I only picked up a paintbrush again properly in 2015 at the age of 28.'

Many people love to draw and paint as children, but as adults become quick to dismiss themselves as 'not being very good' at art. But that shouldn't matter. Indulging a love for any pastime and giving yourself permission to enjoy the process – regardless of the finished result – can be of great therapeutic benefit.

Rebecca describes her experiences: 'Painting is my release. As an adult, there's so much pressure to be something. Painting means I'm at home in comfortable clothes, without make-up, and I can unleash any emotions on to the canvas. I feel like a new person afterwards, even though I then have to clean all the stray paint from the walls and floor.'

Rebecca's work has recently been exhibited in London, Barcelona and York. 'I'm still very bewildered by it all, as I never see it as a job, but a hobby that I adore,' she says. Her advice is to 'give it a go. Focus on how it [your chosen pastime] made you feel when you were younger. Hold on to those childhood moments and relive them.'

You might even find that, as was the case with Rebecca, rediscovering a long-lost passion can be life-changing.

THE WORLD OF YOUR IMAGINATION

Connecting with this childhood version of yourself through visualisation is an easy way to bring some youthful joy into your everyday, even when you don't have time to play. Write an account of a time you remember being absorbed and happy in a game or task as a child. Use the first person and the present tense to really take yourself back to that moment – for example 'I'm sitting on the floor in my bedroom colouring in a drawing, all the pencils are laid out in front of me...' When you've finished, read it back to yourself, then close your eyes and imagine yourself there in that moment of peaceful concentration

....

....

....

....

....

....

....

....

....

....

....

....

....

....

TURN BACK TIME

Looking for inspiration? Start by taking some quiet time to reflect on the things you loved to do as a child. Write down some of your favourite activities

Think about how those memories make you feel. Write down a few key emotions that you associate with these activities

....

....

....

....

....

....

....

Choose one activity that reignites that feeling of pleasure and give it a go. Record how it makes you feel. This could be your new feel-good hobby, one that makes you feel fitter or more creative, while also relaxed and happy. Try indulging your childhood passions – you never know where they might take you

....

....

....

....

....

....

....

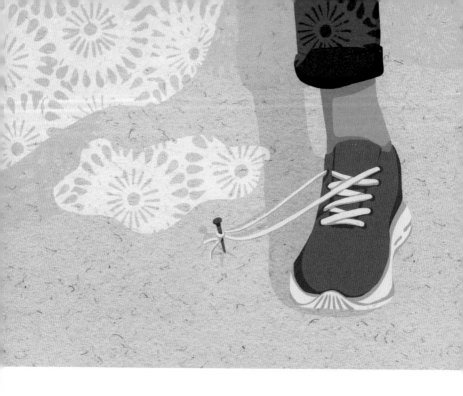

Do life your way

Defying social expectations can be hard, but in the long run it might make you happier

When you're a child, life revolves around your family and community. It can seem like there's one path you're expected to follow, one direction to head in, one way to live. But as you grow into adulthood your world view broadens, and sometimes the life you want doesn't look like what you see around you. What if you want to walk a different path?

It may feel as though a clear route has been set out for you: go to school, then university, get on the career ladder, get married, buy a house, have a family and work until retirement age – or a variation of that rough structure. This may be what your family expects, what you see your friends and peers doing and what you feel you're supposed to do to fit in. For some people, that's great. The course they see laid out in front of them is one they're happy and comfortable to follow.

But, just as each human is unique, there's an individual path they will follow in life. Some are clearly paved and signposted, others have twists, turns and loops. The tricky part is figuring out your path if you don't wish to follow the herd.

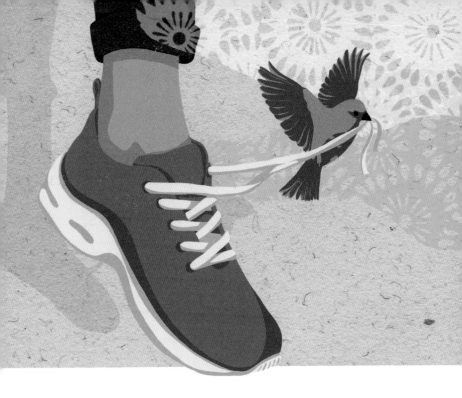

Changing times

Social norms are always evolving, and there have been big changes in recent years. The idea of the nuclear family no longer fits modern society and a job for life is a rarity. According to the Office for National Statistics, the number of people working for themselves in the UK rose from 3.3 million in 2001 to 4.8 million in 2017. The number of opposite-sex couples marrying in England and Wales has been declining since the 1970s and the number of children born each year is falling, too.

There's no set way to define a family anymore. There could be one or several parents of the same or different genders who live together or apart. It might include multiple generations or friends, as well as those with shared DNA.

Similarly, a home no longer has to be made of bricks and mortar and come with a 25-year mortgage. It can be rented, have wheels, float on the water, be self-built or spread across many locations.

The world of work has also changed. The digital revolution means people have different choices to their parents and grandparents. It's now possible to run a global business with a laptop from your kitchen table, a beach or a van.

In her podcast, *There are Other Ways*, Fiona Barrows talks to people living differently. They are united in making a deliberate choice to live how they want to rather than going along with society's expectations. 'Living life a little differently starts with thinking about what it is you really want, and then intentionally designing a life that has the potential to meet it,' says Fiona.

KNOW YOURSELF

Journalling can be a useful way of unearthing thoughts and ideas that might be lying dormant. Begin exploring the kind of life you want by answering the following questions

What are your top three priorities in life?

▶ ....

....

....

▶ ....

....

....

▶ ....

....

....

When are you at your happiest?

....

....

....

....

....

....

....

If you could change one thing about your life as it is now, what would it be?

....

....

....

....

....

....

....

In an ideal world, what would your life be like in three years' time?

....

....

....

....

....

....

....

....

LOOKING FOR INSPIRATION

It can be tricky to imagine the life you want. Finding like-minded people can help you to begin thinking about what you want your life to look like. Joining clubs and interest groups in your area or searching online for people living alternative lifestyles can also trigger ideas.

Look around and you'll most likely see examples of people defying social expectations and living on their own terms – the colleague who turned down promotion because he's content and fulfilled in his current role; the couple in a committed, long-term relationship who choose not to live under the same roof; the friend who resigned from a well-paid career to start her own business; or the neighbour selling up to travel the world with no plan or timescale in place.

Make a list of people you can take inspiration from, they might be friends or family members, or people you've heard or read about, the aim here isn't to make comparisons or to emulate their way of doing things, simply to remind yourself that it can be done

....

....

....

....

....

....

....

....

....

....

....

Please yourself

What if you've dug deep and discovered your desired life only to meet resistance from family and friends?

It can be helpful to remember that when someone criticises or seems unsupportive it often says more about them than it does you. Seeing someone they know decide to change their life and do things differently can prompt them to reassess their own world. They may feel the path you're choosing is a rejection of their life or that you're judging their values. Some will resent the fact that you're brave enough to choose another way that they feel is denied to them. Of course, there will also be kind friends and family who want to shield you from potential disappointment.

If this is the case and you're lacking a supportive, encouraging voice, try to be your own cheerleader. The only person you need permission from is yourself, so fill in the form below to put it in writing

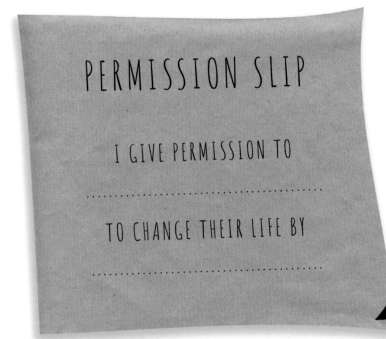

PERMISSION SLIP

I GIVE PERMISSION TO

....

TO CHANGE THEIR LIFE BY

....

My support for this change is informed by my belief that this change/changes will bring them happiness in the following ways

....

....

....

....

....

....

....

....

Let joy lead the way

As you begin to make changes, keep in mind that even during a transformation, there isn't one set path to follow. And it's important to be mindful that radically changing your life on a whim or because you're unhappy with part of yourself may not be the best solution. 'Don't expect to find a magical answer to life, and to suddenly be happy and fulfilled every single day,' cautions Fiona. 'You'll still be you and you'll still be human and have emotions [on] the other side of living life differently. Pay attention to your feelings and what's good and do what brings you satisfaction and joy.'

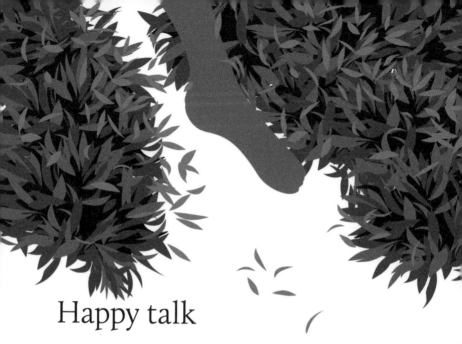

Happy talk

Why it's important to challenge the myths around happiness

Happiness is a loaded word and has different meanings for different people. Some regard it as being all about pleasure – surface-deep, short-lived, fleeting and mainly found through external channels. Others use the word to mean wellbeing – deeper, more meaningful and connected with contentment and ongoing life satisfaction that comes from within. This is what most people want to experience: happiness, joy and contentment that feels bone-deep and is based on finding meaning, human connection and fulfilment in daily life. Let's look at five myths that surround happiness and how to bust them:

1. You're either born happy or you're not. It's not something that you can change

It may surprise you to know that you have more influence over your own happiness than you may have given yourself credit for. Research has found that only 25 to 35 per cent of your potential for happiness is determined by your genes. Whether your parents were the glass-half-full or glass-half-empty types doesn't have a huge impact on how you'll feel. And while your gender, education, age, occupation and geographical location is relevant to how happy you can be, it only accounts for 10 to 15 per cent of your potential.

This means that around 50 per cent – depending on which positive-psychology researcher you talk to – of how happy you can be in your life is determined by you. How you view, react to and act upon events and how you think about and approach life influences how happy you feel. Anyone can increase their base or enduring level of happiness, regardless of age, heritage or circumstances.

2. Happiness is a goal to strive for and reach

You can pursue a moment of happiness and experience it, but once that moment of pleasure is over, you're back to how you felt before. This is known as hedonic adaptation. After your basic needs have been met, money and possessions don't have as great an impact on how happy you feel as you might think. Studies have shown that, although lottery winners experience an initial boost in happiness levels, within a year they return to their original level.

The happiness that doesn't come with rainbows and fireworks but rather with a calmer sense of contentment and lasting joy is an ongoing process that continues throughout a person's lifetime.

3. It's selfish to think about your own happiness

Many people have the view that focusing on your own happiness must mean you're self-centred, narcissistic and downright selfish. If it was all you thought about, then that might be true. If, however, a person is genuinely worried that wanting to be happy reflects an inner selfishness, it's unlikely that they're self-absorbed.

Happy people spread happiness – it truly is contagious (not just a bumper sticker). Social scientists Christakis and Fowler proposed the Three Degrees of Influence theory, which shows the ripple effect of a person's behaviour. Your positive, happy attitude and actions not only rub off on your friends, but also their friends and, in turn, their friends, three people removed from you.

You can see the impact of the ripple effect all around you. Whether it's getting the kids ready for school, in a meeting at work or at the supermarket checkout, if you're feeling happy, you express that directly or indirectly through your words, tone of voice, facial expressions, posture, actions and being, which others pick up on, absorb and can reflect back into the world. Likewise, if you're stressed or in a bad mood, those around you can feel it, too.

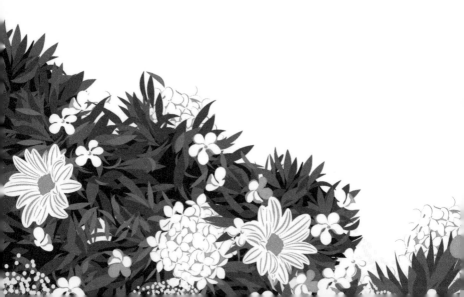

4. To be happy, you can never be sad

While fully in a happy moment, you aren't sad, but that hedonic kind of pleasure isn't a permanent state of being. Eudaemonic wellbeing is about experiencing a range of feelings – not just the positive ones. Denying difficult feelings doesn't guarantee happiness. How well could you experience calm and ease if you'd never felt stress or pressure? Knowing how difficulties and sadness feel means you can experience joy and contentment. It also involves experiencing feelings that you may not have readily associated with happiness, such as purpose, meaning, fulfilment and altruism. Positive-psychology research has found that practising proven methods, such as mindfulness and gratitude, helps increase the happiness you feel and builds resilience. This means you're better able to cope with life's challenges and difficulties and will not necessarily be overwhelmed by the feelings that accompany them.

5. If I let myself be happy something bad is bound to happen

Many people know what it's like to feel utterly happy, completely full of joy, and then a moment later be struck with the fear that something will happen to take away the happy feeling and replace it with pain. US author Brené Brown describes joy as the most terrifying emotion because to experience it you become vulnerable: 'When we lose our tolerance to be vulnerable, joy becomes foreboding.' People think that if they don't let themselves feel too happy, if they keep their joy down to a certain level, that they are protecting themselves from the hurt and pain they could experience when life takes a nosedive. But that's not true. When a loved one is hurt, when redundancy hits, when something goes wrong, you don't feel any less pain because you didn't allow yourself to feel love or happiness with that person or in that job. Keeping happiness at arm's length as a form of protection is misguided – it stops you from living your life to the fullest now, from experiencing true happiness now.

Instead of allowing fear to take over from joy in such moments, practise gratitude. Be thankful for all the things associated with that source of happiness and recognise how grateful you are to know that person, do that job, have whatever's going right go right for you. It challenges fearful feelings while supporting the joy you're experiencing, and research shows that practising gratitude increases and deepens the happiness you feel.

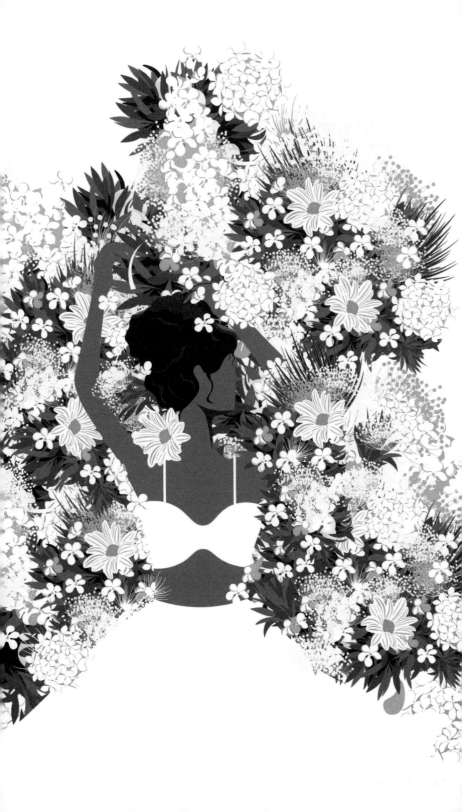

WHAT LIGHTS YOU UP?

Happiness, joy, contentment, wellbeing – whatever word you feel most comfortable using – is something you can create for yourself. It isn't something that requires stuff, nor is it simply a goal to aim for. It's not about denying difficult feelings, you're not selfish to want to feel happy, and by experiencing it you won't make it go away.

When you stop to really think about what makes you happy in your life, you may well find that it isn't the big things like your house, car or holidays. In fact, it isn't the things at all. It's the intangible, seemingly small stuff of life that connects you to others, that has meaning, that lights you up inside.

To appreciate these things more deeply and truly feel the happiness they bring, answer the following five questions

What small acts of kindness could you carry out that would help spread happiness?

....

....

....

....

....

Who are the people in your life that you feel thankful for?

....

....

....

....

....

What everyday aspects of life give you a sense of purpose or meaning?

....

....

....

....

....

What practices (such as mindful meditation or thanksgiving rituals) could you adopt or do more of to cultivate happiness?

....

....

....

....

....

What are the small pleasures that bring you joy each day?

....

....

....

....

....

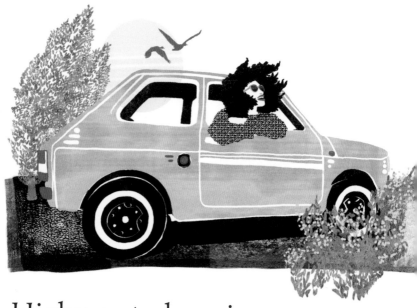

Highway to happiness

Setting short-term targets for change and embracing newness can lead to personal growth

The constant cycle of the seasons is a reminder of how beautiful change can be. Yet the end of each season is also a prelude to letting go for a new phase to occur. If you're feeling stuck or ready for some newness, embracing change can be a route towards a happier life.

Setting out

When contemplating change, it can be difficult to know where to begin. You may have things in mind but feel unsure of how to take the first steps or be disconcerted by the word 'goal'. Surely that's only something you do at work? But you can have fun. It's all about how you decide to approach it.

Olivia Stefanino, coach, speaker and author of *Be Your Own Guru: Personal and Business Enlightenment in Just 3 Days!*, explains: 'When you are looking to make change and set goals, it has to be something you really want for yourself, something you believe in. Even if it's hard work to achieve, if the goal has meaning to you and you own it, you'll keep going.' She adds: 'If you've set the goal because you feel you should do it or only to please or pacify someone else, that's when it gets really tough.'

She suggests that one way of considering what's important to you is to let go of all the things you think you need to do or should do and imagine that you have a magic wand.

MAKE THE CHANGE

Make a note here of how your life would look and feel if you could wave the wand and make it exactly as you want. Olivia recommends giving yourself permission to say what you really want, and don't hold back or think small. Be honest and go for it

....

....

....

....

....

....

....

....

....

....

....

....

....

....

....

....

HOW TO MAKE IT HAPPEN WITHOUT THE MAGIC WAND

When focusing on change, you want to feel motivated and energised by your choices, as opposed to overwhelmed and daunted. Here's one way to make the idea of getting from where you are now to where you really want to be feel possible on a practical level: treat it as though you're taking a car trip to a new destination. You might be excited about the trip, even though you know parts of the journey will be challenging. You've got good reasons for wanting to reach your destination. It's a place you're keen to visit.

As you've not driven this route before, you'll most likely look at a map or review your satnav to ensure you know which direction to go in. You make a note of key roads and any landmarks to indicate progress and reassure yourself that you're heading the right way. There are often myriad ways to get there. You might take the scenic, slow route or the blast-down-the-motorway option. It's your decision, but either way, you can follow these steps:

1. The destination

Begin by defining where you want to end up. You might want to be more creative and start an art project or wish to wear a self-made garment but haven't the first clue how to sew. You've taken that first step to define where you want to go, but what does this look and feel like? Take time to visualise your outcome and how it would feel to achieve it. Picture yourself putting on that new dress you made – the colour, the material, the style. Picture yourself zipping it up and feel your pride.

Your destination. Where are you going? Think about what's important to you

....

....

....

....

....

....

....

....

....

....

....

....

....

....

What will it look and feel like to get there? Do you feel excited, energised and
filled with joy about this trip?

....

....

....

....

....

....

....

....

....

....

2. The route

Even though you have your destination in mind, you know there are many ways to get there. Which ones are you going to take? What new behaviours do you need to introduce? For example, to reach the point of zipping up that dress, you might:

- Embark on sewing lessons or follow instructions online to learn new skills.
- Spend time with a friend who has these skills and ask if they'd be prepared to help.
- Put aside dedicated sewing time.
- Make some simple pieces to get you started.
- Invest in a sewing machine or buy a second-hand one.
- Set up space in your home where you can sew.

Your route. Get specific about the steps to take to reach your destination. What new behaviours do you need to introduce? Remember, there are many ways to get somewhere

....

....

....

....

....

....

....

....

....

....

3. Landmarks
Along the way, you see landmarks indicating your progress:

- You know the basics and are moving on to more advanced techniques.
- You're progressing on to more difficult items.
- You buy the pattern and the fabric for the dress.
- You start to make it.
- You finish it, wear it to an event and can almost hear your satnav making the announcement, 'You have reached your destination'.

You're likely to see tangible results with a creative project – the dress is proof of your achievement. However, it can be helpful to keep a note and write down what it is you want to achieve and how you're progressing, so that you can see your success. Plenty of statistics show that those who have written down their goals achieve greater success.

Your landmarks. Are you on the right road? What will you pass on your way to your destination that indicates you're making good progress?

....

....

....

....

....

....

....

....

4. Timing

Now to timescales... Do you need to reach your destination by a certain date? Perhaps you want to wear the dress to an event that you already have in your diary? You therefore have a deadline. Having a timescale helps you focus. Without one, it's easy to keep telling yourself, 'I'll do it tomorrow'. Some people love long-term goals. They like nothing more than to consider a one-year plan or longer. For others, this can feel like far too much of a commitment. A possible compromise is to set a 90-day timescale. This shorter period gives an opportunity to see real progress. You can start any day you want. Tomorrow, even.

If you wish to create a new habit and commit to something on a daily basis, one technique is to put a cross through the calendar each day you achieve it. It's great when you see a build-up of crosses (you're also less likely to want to buck the trend and have a cross-free day) and it enables you to build a new habit in a relatively easy way.

Your timescale. Set some timescales, perhaps the 90-day suggestion

....

....

....

....

5. Support

Do you want to travel alone or have someone along for the ride? If you opt for a co-driver, it could be someone you know to be supportive or a friend who's also trying to set some goals. Knowing you'll be sharing progress is a great way to keep that momentum going.

Your support team. Are you going it alone or do you want a co-driver? Sharing your progress with someone else can be an added incentive to keep going

....

....

....

....

....

6. Diversions

All trips have an element of the unknown, no matter how much you plan ahead. You may get delayed or have to take a diversion. If that happens, go easy on yourself, give yourself space and think it over. To prevent diversions from sending you off course completely, it can be useful to anticipate some of the challenges you might face in advance.

Your possible diversions. Think about the obstacles you might face as you progress along your planned route. Are there any contingency plans you can put in place to help you keep moving?

....

....

....

....

....

....

....

....

....

....

....

....

And Olivia has one final piece of advice: 'When you're contemplating what you want, think about what you'd want for your own child or a best friend. You'd want the very best for them, so apply the same approach to yourself. Set your own plans in motion from a place of love. You're far more likely to succeed if you set out to do something that brings you joy, fills you with excitement and comes from the heart.'

Sacred sunshine

Throughout history, the sun has been revered by many cultures as a giver of life, as well as light and heat. It's central to many spiritual beliefs, celebrated in customs and festivals around the world and, in more recent times, has been scientifically proven to make people feel good

The worship of nature can appear obscure to modern city dwellers, but honouring a deep connection to the Earth is something many groups, including those who follow shamanism, paganism, theism and animism, have been doing for many thousands of years.

Ancient Eastern texts such as *The Upanishads* (composed between 800 and 400 BCE) repeatedly reference nature and its forces and elements, regarding them as gods and goddesses. Indian civilisation is said to be born of the Aryan and Indus Valley cultures. The Aryans brought with them gods, including Agni, Indra, Vayu, Ratri, Usha, Surya and Yama (respectively fire, the storm, wind, night, dawn, the sun and death). Their powerful god, Surya, also known as Savitri, is thought of as the giver of life and enlightenment.

The rising sun in India is especially connected to this sense of importance and sacredness, with the stillness of the morning light conducive to meditation. The sun is seen as the dispeller of darkness and ignorance, and has the ability to empower knowledge and a harmonious life. The vast and rich Indian epic poem, *The Mahabharata*, opens with a hymn based upon Surya, noting 'him' as the 'Eye of the universe, soul of all existence, origin of all life, goal of the Samkhyas and Yogis' and as a symbol for freedom and liberation.

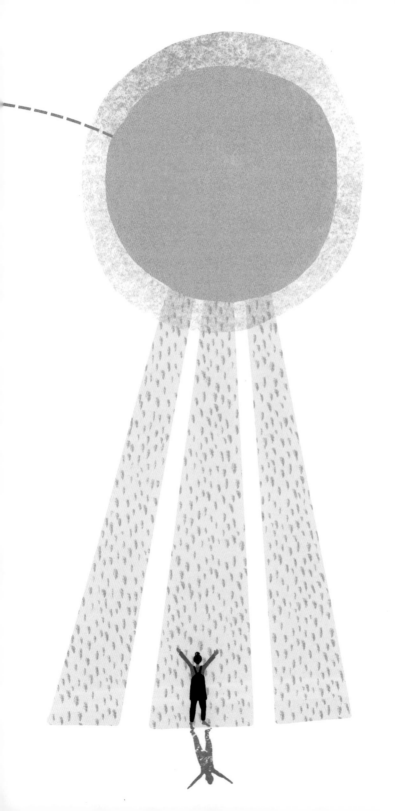

Morning mantras

Early-morning hymns dedicated to the sun are plentiful throughout Indian culture, and most speak of the triumph of good over evil, wisdom over ignorance, darkness over light, and life over death. *The Rig Veda*, compiled by seers or ancient and knowledgeable sages, gives many passages to the adoration of the sun, and written among its pages are verses such as:

'Thou goest across the sky's broad place
Meeting the days with rays, O Sun,
And watching generations pass.'

Also from *The Rig Veda*, the Gayatri mantra is one of the most well-known Eastern mantras chanted in western yoga classes today, dedicated to the sun as giver of life:

'om bhūr bhuvah svah
tatsaviturvarenyam
bhargo devasyadhīmahi
dhiyo yo nah pracodayāt'

Douglas Brooks, a scholar of Hinduism and south-Asian languages, translates this as:

'The eternal, earth, air, heaven
That glory, that resplendence of the sun
May we contemplate the brilliance of that light
May the sun inspire our minds'

SUN WORSHIP

Developing your own morning sun ritual can be a positive way to start the day. Using your own words to give thanks can make mantras more meaningful. Try writing your own hymn, prayer or simple statement of gratitude for the sun's rays

....

....

....

....

....

....

....

....

....

....

....

....

....

....

....

....

Happy days

Today, the sun continues to be worshipped across the world. In the UK, around 30,000 people visit the prehistoric monument of Stonehenge in Wiltshire to mark the summer solstice. Although its origins are debated, aspects of the monument line up perfectly with the summer and winter solstice sunrise and allow for a communion with the ever-changing light.

Other parts of the world give just as much importance to the summer solstice. The pagan custom of lighting bonfires is practised in parts of Greece, France and Norway, while Sweden's midsummer festival is one of the biggest events in the country's holiday calendar – Midsummer's Eve rivals Christmas in importance and tradition. In northern Sweden, the sun doesn't set during midsummer, providing plenty of time to enjoy nature. With the landscape in full bloom, flowers are gathered and fashioned into floral crowns for girls to harness the magic of midsummer and ensure good health throughout the year, with everyone coming together for dancing and feasting on pickled herring, new potatoes and schnapps.

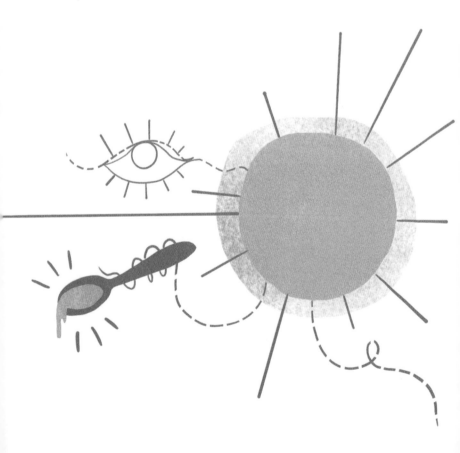

SUN CELEBRATION

Make a list of some of your own summertime traditions. Getting together with friends and family for a picnic or doing an annual walk or swim can all be forms of ritual

➤ ....
....

➤ ....
....

➤ ....
....

➤ ....
....

➤ ....
....

➤ ....
....

➤ ....
....

➤ ....
....

➤ ....
....

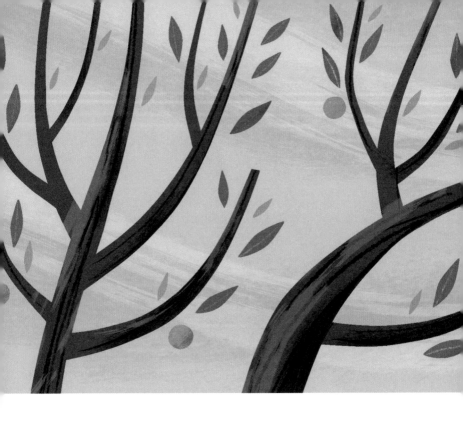

Branching out

In our modern world, more and more of us are becoming detached from nature. But there's an easy way to reconnect with the Earth and lift our spirits at the same time – make friends with trees

In the hubbub of modern society, trees can often appear little more than great statues lining our streets and avenues, passive observers of the teeming life below. But throughout history they have played a vital role in our psychic and cultural development, and they continue to enrich our lives, lift our spirits, feed our souls and sustain our planet. They also, according to recent research, emit vibrations that can have positive benefits on our health and happiness. Perhaps the often-derided tree-huggers have been right all along.

Historical roots
But where does our history with trees begin? The mark or symbol of the hawthorn was present in the runic alphabets of ancient British tribes; in Wales, the yew symbolises the immortality of the soul, a belief originating from Celtic druids; sycamores are considered part of the scenery, where the soul of the

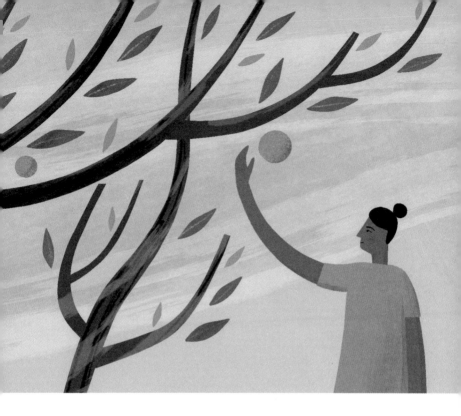

deceased finds peace in the ancient Egyptian *Book of the Dead*, while in Greek mythology, the trees of the Dodona Grove, which were built into the prow of the ship *Argo*, retained their gifts of speech and prophecy and guided Jason and his crew on their voyage.

The life and flow of trees also appear in the Germanic Hulders, the Norwegian Yggdrasil, and they are significant in many religions including Hinduism, Judaism and Christianity. In modern-day western society, the branches of trees are woven into the cultural landscape: Robin Hood, who lived in Sherwood Forest with his band of Merry Men; poet William Blake's visionary oak sapling filled with angel wings; Paul McCartney's *Little Willow*; and the paintings of the likes of David Hockney, Georgia O'Keeffe and Henry Moore, to name a few.

Of course, as well as being talked to, worshipped, painted and sung about, trees have always been climbed, as is reflected in this excerpt from Robert Frost's poem, *Birches*:

'I'd like to go by climbing a birch tree,
And climb black branches up a snow-white trunk
Toward heaven, till the tree could bear no more,
But dipped its top and set me down again.
That would be good both going and coming back.
One could do worse than be a swinger of birches.'

ODE TO AN OAK

Expressing appreciation and gratitude for the things that bring happiness can enhance the good feelings still further. Try writing your own poem or thank-you note to your favourite tree. You might like to include some details about its branches, bark and leaves or perhaps describe the way it changes with the seasons

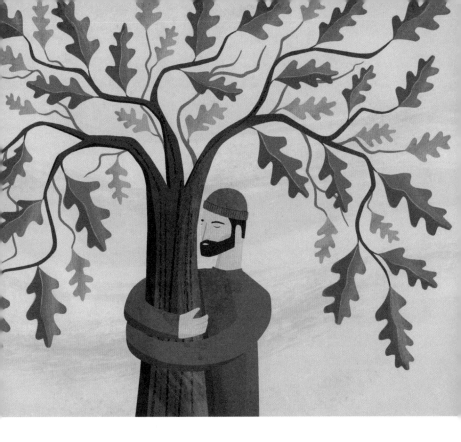

Good vibrations

For most of us, climbing trees stops when we become adults. Yet new research suggests we would do well to continue our physical contact with them long after we've left our childhood behind. This needn't mean climbing them, of course. There are easier ways to maintain the connection. Tree-hugging, long considered the primary activity of hippies and conservationists, may provide some previously undiscovered health benefits. Aside from the physical and psychological benefits of taking a 30-minute walk in nature, which has been proven to help alleviate depression and improve memory and creativity, actual contact with the trees you walk among may be beneficial. It's all to do with the vibrations they emit. A recent experiment demonstrated that drinking a glass of water treated with a 10Hz vibration changes your blood coagulation rates immediately. As everything is made of vibrating energy, so, too, are trees, and the benefits of tree-hugging are, in part, to do with their vibrational properties and patterns. Ultimately, however, it is about feeling connected with nature.

Luckily, there are many trees out there to hug – in urban areas in particular they represent calming groves of respite – and they play a vital role in life on Earth, releasing oxygen and absorbing carbon dioxide. For us, living in a man-made environment, they are the primary means of staying connected with the Earth, the seasons and the wheel of life.

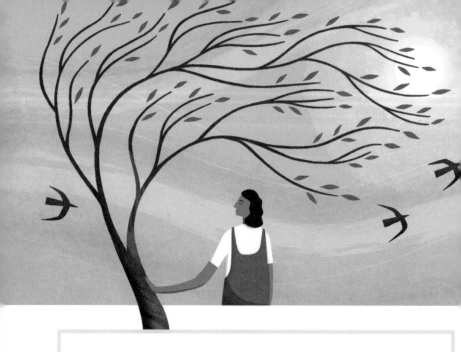

POWER OF CONNECTION

Follow these simple steps to start tree-hugging

- Find yourself a quiet forest, park or woodland area.

- Try to be present as you walk among the trees: listen to the rustle of the leaves in the wind, take in the smells around you, feel the different bark textures with your hands and find a tree you feel comfortable with.

- Encircle the tree with your arm and gently, pressing your forehead to the trunk, give the tree a good squeeze.

- Try to imagine the energy you are absorbing. Imagine how old the tree is, how long it has been on Earth, how much wisdom it has absorbed. You can even talk to your tree – it won't judge you.

- When you feel ready, turn around so that your back is against the tree, and put your arms around it, behind you. Feel the way it supports you as you face the world.

- When you have finished, you might like to thank the tree.

SOLID ROOTS

Although deforestation has destroyed many forests and rainforests, there are still incredible places to visit where you'll find some magical old trees. Here are just a few

Sherwood National Forest
This forest in Nottinghamshire is that of the medieval legend of Robin Hood. In the nearby village of Edwinstowe stands Major Oak, the oak tree fabled to have sheltered Robin Hood and his Merry Men.

General Sherman
Named after US Civil War General William Tecumseh Sherman, this is a giant sequoia situated in California's spectacular Sequoia National Park. The largest known single-stem tree on the planet, it stands at just over 274ft tall and is estimated to be between 2,000 and 3,000 years old.

Banagher Glen
Local legend has it that Banagher Glen in Northern Ireland, one of the few forests untouched by deforestation, is where St Patrick trapped the last snake in the country. The forest, full of oak, hazel, hawthorn, holly and ash, is set in a ravine and is the perfect backdrop to view wildlife and maybe catch sight of the snake!

El Árbol del Tule
The circumference of this giant Montezuma cypress, which towers over the little church of Santa María del Tule, in Oaxaca, Mexico, is thought to be the widest tree trunk on the planet, with estimates varying from 130ft to 170ft. Local legend says it was planted by an Aztec storm god 2,000 years ago.

The Bodhi Tree
In Bodh Gaya, India, this fig tree remains an important place of pilgrimage as is believed to be the tree under which Siddhartha Gautama achieved enlightenment 2,500 years ago. Buddhist texts describe how, afterwards, the Buddha gazed up at the tree in gratitude, eyes unblinking, for a week.

'The clearest way into the universe
is through a forest wilderness'

John Muir

Essence of life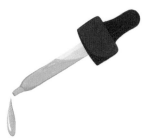

Flowers are perhaps the most delightful and uplifting expression of the natural world. They brighten up surroundings, inspire art and poetry and help to convey feelings when the right words are hard to find. But flowers have an even greater gift – the healing power to restore mental and emotional harmony through their essence

Flower essences are nature's remedies. They work on a subtle energetic level – in a similar way to homeopathy – to create a balancing effect on the mind and emotions.

Flowers have long been known for their benefits on wellbeing, and many ancient cultures recognised their therapeutic qualities and curative powers:

- In the 12th century, Abbess Hildegard von Bingen, known as the mother of German botany, collected dew from flowers to treat health imbalances.
- In the 16th century, Paracelsus, a Swiss healer, botanist and mystic, also studied how flowers heal emotional disharmony.
- In the early 1930s, through the pioneering work of prominent English physician Dr Edward Bach, flower essences became more widely known as a natural system of healing.

The roots of rescue

Edward abandoned his successful medical practice to focus on finding simple, natural remedies for wellbeing. After extensive research, studies and field trips, he found that the dew collected from a flower in sunlight possessed a special healing quality. His recognition that each flower had specific properties with a positive resonance on the emotions led to the birth of the Bach Flower Remedies, including the popular Bach Rescue Remedy.

There are now a plethora of flower remedies worldwide.

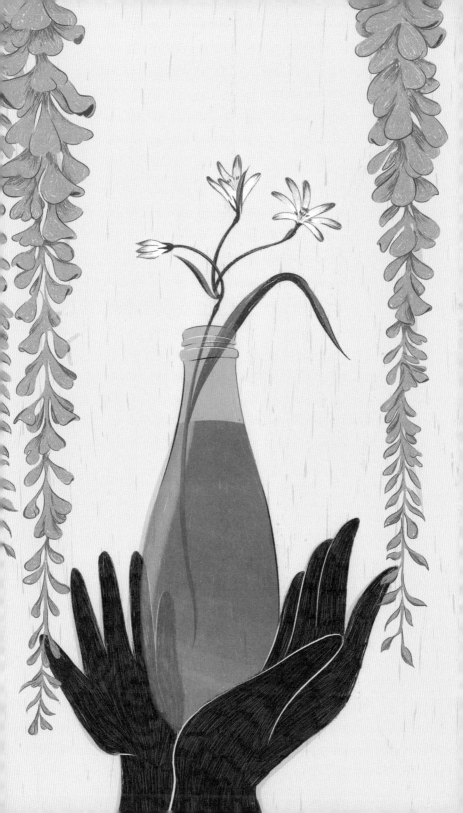

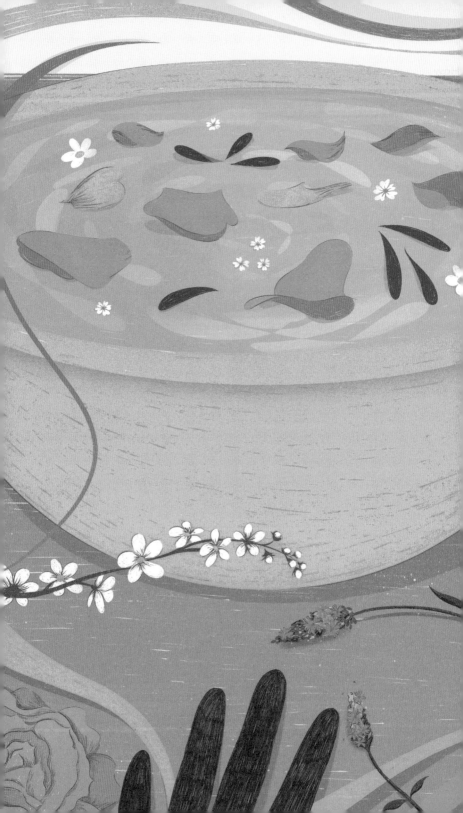

How they're made

Most of the liquid remedies are prepared in the same three-step process:

- The plant or tree blossom is placed in a bowl of distilled water and left in the sun for several hours so that the healing essence or energy imprint of the flower is transferred into the water.
- The blossom is then removed, and the essence-infused liquid is preserved, usually in brandy.
- The preserved essence is diluted with water to create the remedy, which can be dropped straight onto the tongue.

Helping people blossom

Jackie Stewart is a soul alchemist and advanced-practitioner member of the British Flower and Vibrational Essences Association and has been prescribing flower essences professionally since 1999. 'Taking essences shines the light of awareness on parts of you that call to be seen,' she says. 'Every time you take essences, you are transforming the energy of emotions and beliefs that hold you back. You'll notice things beginning to change for the better in subtle – and sometimes not so subtle – ways. You might have more clarity or find it easier to make decisions. People say it's like the parts that aren't their true nature fall away and it becomes easier to make positive changes.'

These changes can have a beneficial impact on all aspects of wellbeing. Stefan Ball, from the Bach Centre in Wallingford, Oxfordshire, says: 'Dr Bach's system is aimed purely at emotional states and personality characteristics, so the only important consideration is: "How do we feel today?" And I mean emotionally. Physical or medical issues are only relevant in so far as they lead us to ask how we feel about them.'

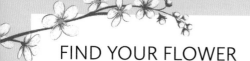

FIND YOUR FLOWER

What's reassuring about flower remedies is that they are safe and not intended to replace medical treatment but to support it. If you're not sure which flower essences will be beneficial, or if you feel that you need support on your healing journey, it is best to consult a qualified flower-remedies practitioner. You can, however, work with flower essences on your own. Consult the panel below to find out some of the properties of popular flowers, but first ask yourself the following questions to help hone your choice:

What are the core issues you want to focus on?

....

....

....

....

What change would make the biggest difference to your life?

....

....

....

....

....

What qualities would you most like to embody and awaken within yourself?

....

....

....

....

What are the core beliefs, emotions or dynamics that trip you up – lack of confidence or motivation, indecision, being unable to express yourself?

....

....

....

....

....

Are there any patterns of behaviour that you'd most like to reset?

....

....

....

....

....

Positive petals

In these times, where it's easy to be overwhelmed by busy schedules, technology, work and the state of the world, taking flower essences is an act of self-care.

'There is a great deal of negative emotional energy in the world, and also more distance from nature,' says Stefan. 'So a system based on simple flowers, on what Dr Bach called "the clean, pure, beautiful agents of nature" – and that works, above all, to dispel negatives like hatred, scorn, anger and fear – must have a special part to play. It requires moments of introspection, quiet and self-examination, and every time we take our chosen drops from the bottle, that, too, is a little oasis of reflection time built into the day.'

FEEL-GOOD FLORA

Honeysuckle
For letting go
Are you struggling to let go of the past? Do you feel nostalgic for happier times? Honeysuckle flower remedy is excellent for those who find it difficult to be present because they are focused on the past. The remedy will help dissolve the intense feelings that come with regret, sadness, homesickness, divorce, bereavement or loss of any kind. If you feel that happiness can only be found in the past, honeysuckle will help you accept and let go of nostalgia, so that you can begin to feel joy in the present moment.

Hornbeam
For mental vitality
Do you drink several cups of coffee in the morning to help you get going? Do you feel like you just don't have enough strength to carry out everyday tasks? If you're feeling mentally tired, even after a good night's sleep, and find it takes you a while to feel motivated, try hornbeam. This remedy acts as a strengthener for mind and body, and encourages a feeling of vitality to ward off staleness and procrastination.

Agrimony
For anxiety and bottled-up emotions
If you're putting on a cheerful face to the outside world, but feel like you're going through hell on the inside, agrimony could help you express your true feelings, while restoring inner peace and harmony.

Gentian
For discouragement after a setback
This remedy is for when you're feeling downhearted or slightly pessimistic and are struggling to see a positive outcome. Gentian will give you a gentle lift to raise your spirits. If you find yourself undone and dejected by seemingly small hiccups or are a slave to your inner doubter, you might find that gentian helps you to regain your confidence and sense of your own ability.

Clematis
For lack of concentration and mindfulness
If you're a daydreamer with your head in the clouds and think more about the future rather than being in the present, clematis can bring you into the here and now and help you to concentrate. This remedy is also beneficial for creative people with over-active imaginations who find it difficult to be attentive, grounded and 'in the moment'.

Vervain
For overenthusiasm and perfectionism
Are you a perfectionist? Perhaps a bit fanatical? Do you struggle to listen to and consider other people's viewpoints? Do you throw yourself into everything you do with far too much effort that only leaves you drained? Vervain will help you to relax and realise that it's not up to you to fix everything or change things or other people to suit your ideals or beliefs. This remedy helps you to restore balance and encourages you to enjoy life without always feeling the need to be active and perfect.

Pine
For guilt or self-blame
Pine is good if you tend to blame yourself and feel guilty for a situation that's not your fault. You may say 'sorry' a lot, even when there is no need to do so. This remedy helps you to restore a positive sense of self-worth, to know when you're not to blame, to acknowledge any faults without dwelling on them, and to put right any wrongs where possible knowing that you have done your best.

Star of Bethlehem
For shock
For any traumatic situation, distress, accident or unexpected bad news, star of Bethlehem is an effective remedy. If this essence is given immediately after experiencing shock, it will greatly assist in recovery. This remedy is also effective for people experiencing loss or emptiness after losing a loved one and can bring a sense of much-needed comfort.

Please note that all flower remedies are complementary to wellbeing and you should consult a professional health practitioner if you have any medical concerns.

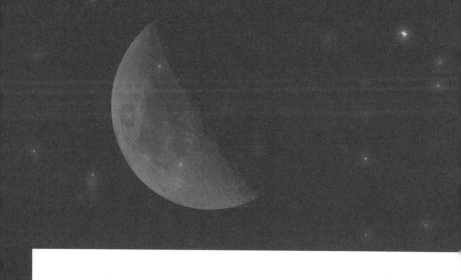

By the light of the Moon

Could tuning into lunar cycles be the key to a happier life?

Tick-tock, tick-tock, tick-tock – does the clock on the wall say you're late for a doctor's appointment, need to be at work or only have hours left to file your accounts? Maybe you're on schedule, in the GP's waiting room, at your desk and up to date with your finances. Either way, life can feel as though it's being dictated by 'wall time'. But this hasn't always been the case. Our ancestors were guided by the phases of the Moon, which offer a more cyclical and, some argue, intuitive way of living – a natural calendar that promotes self-awareness and a less stressful means of navigating life's changes.

Reawakening to nature's clock
While mechanised, chronological accuracy has many advantages – trains (sometimes) running to timetables, for example – its precise, repetitive pattern doesn't necessarily encourage the intuitive reflection or self-awareness that can help you live a happy life. It can also contribute to feelings of stress and tiredness.

The functional rhythm of wall time does suit some people, but if you find it unsatisfying, you might find listening to your inner clock and developing a different relationship with time more fulfilling. How do you do this? Next time you have a few minutes to yourself of an evening, go outside and look up into the infinite expanse of the night sky. The chances are you'll see an old friend – someone who soothes and calms, who has been waiting for you to feel their presence in your life: the oldest and best timekeeper of them all – the Moon.

The gravitational pull of this celestial body controls the Earth's tidal patterns. It also influences many of the planet's organisms and life forms whose behaviour and mating patterns run in perfect synchronicity with the lunar cycles.

Turning the clocks back

Our ancestors had an intuitive and intimate relationship with their revered Moon. Archaeology shows that people have been marking out the lunar phases for 26,000 years, and written records from ancient civilisations indicate they believed they controlled, fertility, seasonal growth and crops. Important ceremonies were also timed to coincide with the different phases of the Moon. With the industrial and technological advancement of society, much of this celestial knowledge has fallen by the wayside. But could personal wellbeing and peace be found by realigning one's thought patterns, life path and calendar with the phases of the tranquil, pearlescent Moon? What if society rediscovered and reconnected with nature's own tempo?

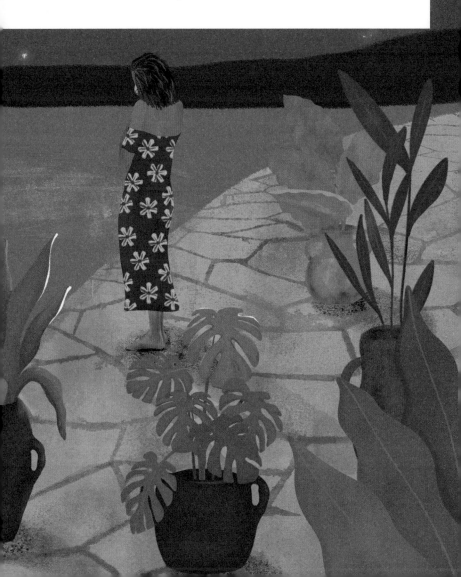

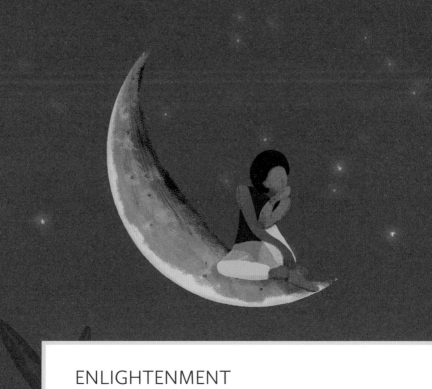

ENLIGHTENMENT IN THE MOONLIGHT

The Moon was important for many ancient civilisations

- Ancient India – sages held that the Moon controlled the Earth's water, and would advise people to refrain from various commitments on important Moon days and instead relax their minds and devote time to spiritual pursuits.

- Buddhists also place great significance on the full Moon. Records suggest that all the important episodes in the Buddha's life – including his birth, renunciation, enlightenment, first teachings and death – happened on full-Moon days.

- Ancient Greek and Roman philosophers, such as Aristotle and Pliny the Elder, regarded the Moon as a mirror to the world. In a similar way, the mind can also be seen as a mirror, receiving and reflecting the goings-on in the surrounding world. Each month, as the light of the Moon grows, so the individual mind changes and responds to reflect what is happening around it.

Discover Moon time

Like life itself, the Moon is constantly changing, going through different phases. Accepting that you are at one with the universe can help you to cope with transitions in life, even difficult and challenging ones. Practising mindfulness on specific phase days can help cultivate an awareness of this synchronicity between mind and Moon. And by consciously viewing this celestial neighbour as a timing device and using it to help direct your mind into a busy or a calm phase, you can find your own version of enlightenment.

It's easy to follow this ancient calendar by simply tracking the Moon's visibility in the night sky. There are four distinct phases of the Moon every month, each one lasting approximately seven days.

4 phases = 4 lunar weeks = 28 days = one lunar cycle.

Each lunar week will present you with a different face in the sky. They are called the new Moon, first quarter, full Moon and last quarter. For 14 days (from new Moon to full Moon), the light on the Moon's face is growing. This is the waxing stage. Then, for the next 14 days (from full Moon to new Moon), the light on the face gradually disappears. This is the waning stage. Each of the four lunar weeks has its own qualities that offer creative inspiration. By channelling them, it's possible to live a calmer, more reflective life.

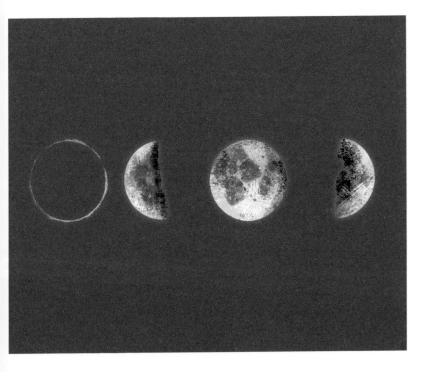

1. New Moon

The Moon is not visible. It sits between the Sun and the Earth with the dark side facing us. But soon the Moon starts to grow, passing through the thin, crescent phase, during which the bright side (right) will increase. This is the seeding phase, when you consciously create an intention.

Write down your hopes and wishes for the month ahead

....

....

....

....

....

....

....

....

....

....

....

....

....

....

....

....

....

2. First quarter

The entire right side of the Moon is illuminated and looks like a semi-circle. It continues to grow as it passes through the gibbous phase, which means that more than one half is visible but it's still not full. This is the sprouting phase, when the things you started at new Moon become more easily perceived in consciousness. This creates some motivational tension – a bit of a push gets you somewhere.

Write down some specific ideas for how to work towards your goals

....

....

....

....

....

....

....

....

....

....

....

....

....

....

....

3. Full Moon

The Moon is fully illuminated and shows its entire face. This is the peak of the cycle. It is the flowering phase, when you are fully illuminated and what might have been hidden before is in the light for all to see. This is when mindfulness helps to create a balance and bring about the manifestation of your ideas.

Write down all the things you are thankful for

....

....

....

....

....

....

....

....

....

....

....

....

....

....

4. Last quarter

The light is diminishing, passing through the disseminating phase, when the dark side of the Moon appears on the right side and, each night, the light diminishes towards the left side. This is the fruiting phase, when you get to enjoy the benefits of what's been created. It's the time to integrate and learn from the wisdom accrued by the experiences of the past 21 days.

Write down your reflections on how far you have come, including any barriers you came across and how you overcame them

....

....

....

....

....

....

....

....

....

....

....

....

....

....

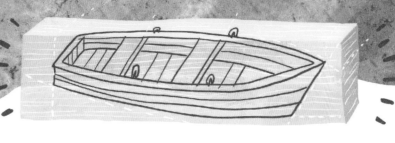

Opportunity knocks

Single-minded aims have their purpose, but sometimes, acting on a whim can lead you to a life-enhancing change of direction – if you let your inner compass be your guide

Stepping out

If you gave a young child a cheap video camera to play with, would you imagine that it would put them on the path to an Oscar? British animator and film-maker Nick Park has much to thank for his series of Wallace & Gromit films, but his father's gift is at the top of the list. Few life paths can be so clear cut. Charting a new direction in life can be a real challenge, but people have been finding alternative paths to take for a very long time.

'The journey of a thousand miles begins with a single step'

More than 2,000 years ago, this was the answer of Lao Tzu, the father of Taoist philosophy. It's a beguilingly simple statement, but profound. You need only start with the first step. Nothing stopped you from taking the first wobbly step around your first birthday. That was a milestone. And, not so long after, you were thinking some extraordinary thoughts: playing with imaginary friends ('I can win'), fleeing the monster ('I can escape') or pretending to be a plane ('I can fly'). The infant brain has many more synapses than the adult one, open to a multitude of connections and able to indulge in what's called 'counterfactual thinking'. That free play with your imagination took you to magical places. You lived adventurously, health and safety permitting. If you were lucky, it sowed seeds for the future.

Finding inspiration

At three or four, a young boy was playing in his front garden, building what he might now call an amphitheatre with a few wooden bricks, when a passerby said, 'Give me one of those bricks'. He couldn't argue. What happened next filled him with horror. The stranger took out a knife and began whittling away chunks of the boy's precious brick. In no time at all, he handed back not a brick, but a boat. Awestruck, the boy ran inside to show his mother. The stranger had disappeared, but the memory remained. Little wonder that, many steps later, the boy-turned-man found himself teaching children to turn clay into all manner of creations.

'Life isn't about finding yourself; life is about creating yourself'

This was George Bernard Shaw's interesting insight. Those moments of epiphany can happen at any time. Writer and dragonfly ambassador Ruary Mackenzie Dodds took time out from a stressful job to walk along a canal when a dragonfly landed on his shirt. It was the first time he'd ever looked at one close up. He was so electrified by this 'little piece of flying crystal' that he went on to establish Europe's first dragonfly sanctuary and is recognised as one of Britain's greatest living naturalists.

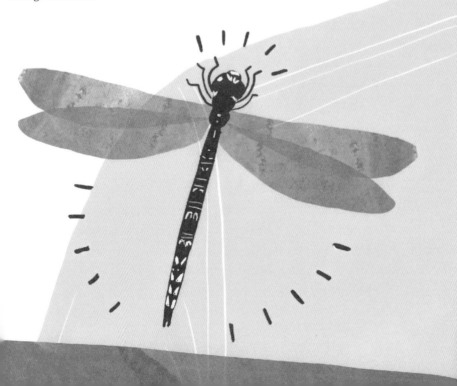

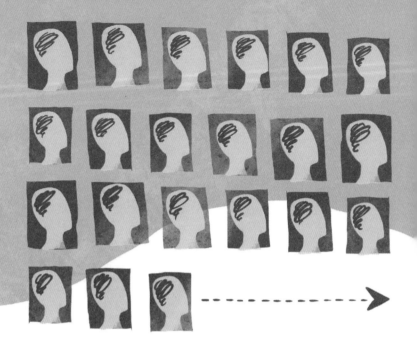

Taking action

Varying a normal routine is a vital first step to change. 'If you do what you've always done, you'll get what you've always gotten' goes the ungainly saying. Cognitive behaviour therapists assert that it takes only 21 repetitions of a behaviour to make it a habit. Plenty of scope for habit-forming there.

'We prefer existing states of affairs over alternate realities just because of the mere fact of their being'

So wrote science journalist Matthew Hutson. Somehow, you have to break out of the familiar, even if it means forming new habits. One of the most powerful ways is to harness your emotional intelligence and the intuition that goes with it. When lyricist Tim Rice got lost while driving in a city, he happened to catch the first few minutes of a radio programme about Eva Peron. That was enough to excite his imagination. Emotional satnav took him to *Evita*. Listening to that inner voice and acting on it helps you to trust the guidance you receive.

The most profound discoveries often follow from happy accidents that initiate actions you might not otherwise have thought of. Where would people be without the accidental invention of sticky notes (after a researcher mistakenly created a very weak adhesive when he meant to make a strong one)? Single-minded aims have their place, of course, but stuff happens. It can be very hard to think so at the time, but a setback can be the shock you need to redirect your life in a more fruitful direction.

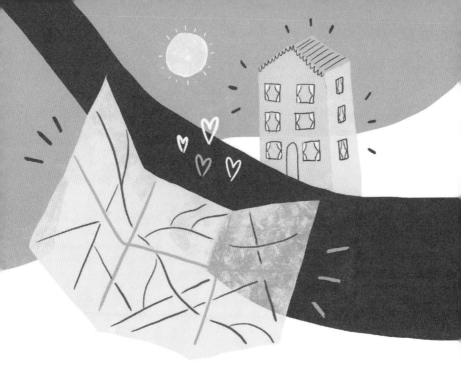

A different path

A simple goodwill gesture can reap unexpected rewards. Take the bookseller who stepped outside his shop when he saw a woman poring over a map. Helping her find the way, he found his way to her heart and a happy marriage.

'There is a process of responsive evocation; the world calling forth something in one that in turn calls forth something in the world'

Writer and psychiatrist Iain McGilchrist insists that people are often more connected with the world out there than they think. Putting yourself in unfamiliar situations opens up new opportunities.

Taking a different route to the park one day, a man came across a three-storey doll's house that had been put out with the rubbish. It had curtains at every window and pictures on the walls and was ripe for a recycling makeover. The man repainted it, patched up the wallpaper, fitted a missing canopy to a balcony, replaced a door and found model characters to occupy each new studio apartment, together with furniture and floor coverings. The whole project was great fun and the house presently graces his granddaughter's playroom. Now he is charged with writing the stories of each resident family.

It's just one example of what may unfold when you take the road less travelled and simply open your eyes. Take all your senses for a walk and there's no knowing where they will lead.

TAKE TIME TO REFLECT

Think about the aspects of your life that you feel most proud of and write about any key moments that set the spark alight and led you in that direction

....

....

....

....

....

....

....

....

....

....

....

....

....

....

....

....

....

....

FIND INSPIRATION

Are there any first steps that you've been too afraid to take? Make a list of some life goals that you've yet to realise and note down beside each how you might break out of the familiar to start working towards them

....

....

....

....

....

....

....

....

....

....

....

....

....

....

....

....

....

....

....

> 'To practise any art, no matter how well or badly, is a way to make your soul grow. So do it.'

Kurt Vonnegut

Creativity: feel the flow

How to get the spark back when inspiration is failing you

Creativity has a mystique. It's not something that can be easily pinned down. If you have a creative job or hobby, it can feel like an essence that brings joy, but it can just as mysteriously slip through your fingers. Finding that drive again can be tricky, but an unexpected dip in inspiration doesn't have to mean waiting around for the spark to return. There are plenty of ways to encourage that innovative engine to run once more and get you back in that happy state of flow.

When creativity is part of your everyday life, it's crucial to understand it. As a quality or ability, it isn't a basic human trait or something ever-flowing in an artist's mind. That's a nice idea, but it's not the reality. It seems to come and go as it pleases. There will be highs and lows. A slump isn't the end of the world or a sign of a declining skill, so don't be tempted to hit your head against the wall or give up on projects – that will release only some of the frustration. It's best to accept the moment for what it is. Let go of the desire to try to control creativity and it will become easier to navigate any slumps that come your way.

Find your spark

Contrary to the suggestion of some headlines, there's little concrete evidence of a specific way to increase creativity. There's no magical method to live at a constant creative peak – everyone does their best and finds what brings on their own inspiration.

Here's the thing: just accepting the fact that you're in a slump won't suddenly make you feel creative again. It's important to acknowledge this because you may be there for a while. You have to push through the lows to get to the highs. It might be the case that the low isn't the result of something you've done. Sometimes, the best advice is just to keep chugging along. It may not be the fastest route, but it'll get you through.

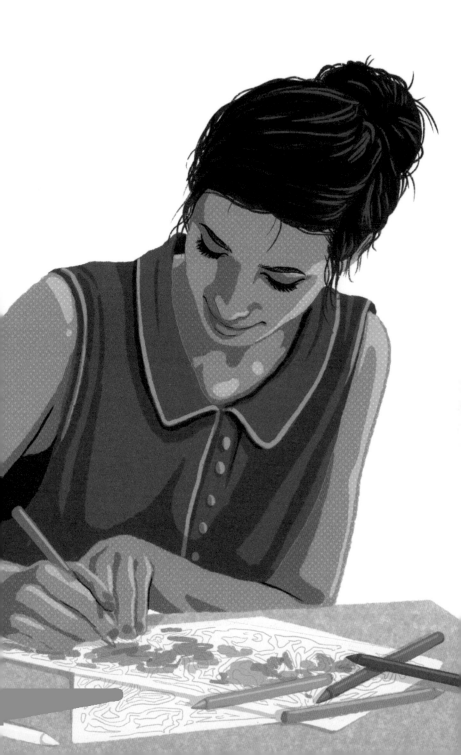

Express your emotions

When searching for something new, don't always look for razor-sharp focus. Rather, seek a state where the mind is open to many ideas and allow yourself to think beyond your regular patterns. Psychologist Eddie Harmon-Jones shared his studies with *Harvard Business Review* magazine about the link between creativity and emotions. He found that, for creativity, you should look for emotions that create a 'low motivational intensity'. In other words, a feeling where you're searching for something, digging deep, but not too focused on the exact details of any one thing. These emotions leave you more open to new ideas and give you the motivation to seek out more unusual thoughts.

That might seem clear-cut, but emotions are complicated. Few people have a single emotion in any given moment. It's usually a mixture of several feelings and reactions to your mind and surroundings. Finding an ideal state for creativity may seem impossible, but there are ways to keep track of how you're feeling and what's causing some of those emotions.

Close your eyes for a moment and take three deep breaths to relax the body and focus the mind. Gradually allow the emotions you're feeling in this moment to rise to the surface. Write down each emotion that you can identify and make a note of anything that might be behind those emotions

UNDERSTAND THE WORKINGS

Journalling over the course of a week is an effective way to catalogue this, and it allows you to look back and discover any patterns. If re-reading entries identifies a distraction, such as watching cute animal videos instead of focusing on work, you can begin to plan how to make your emotions work more effectively for you. Pair your low-motivation activities with the beginning of the brainstorming process – bring on those cat clips! Then channel your high-attention and motivational activities when you need to hunker down and work with details to get things done. It can help to be honest with yourself about what works for you and what doesn't.

Make a list of the things that help trigger creativity

....

....

....

....

....

And the things that tend to hamper creativity

....

....

....

....

When it comes to creativity, low- and high-motivational periods are needed in the same way as varying emotions. Work with these emotions in different ways, but don't ignore them.

Finding ways to focus on creativity is important, but there are also times when it can be detrimental. If you're mid-project, focused yet feeling drained, don't push aside how you feel, either psychologically or physically. Self-care is important now. Take a break, meditate or call a friend to talk through your feelings.

THINK YOUR WAY THROUGH

Sometimes, giving yourself time to identify the nature of the creative block can help you get past it. Try these three steps to return to a state of joyful creativity:

1. Take stock of where you are with the process

Is there anything standing in your way? What's missing from this situation?

....

....

....

....

....

If you're at the start of a project, what's your inspiration?

....

....

....

....

....

What else is taking up your time or distracting you? How can this be remedied?

....

....

....

....

....

Is there an absence of structure? How could you break things down into manageable chunks?

....

....

....

....

....

....

What support do you need to find the discipline to sit down and plough through until the end?

....

....

....

....

....

....

What impact is your environment having? It may be too cluttered, too open or maybe you just need a change of scene

....

....

....

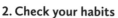

2. Check your habits

Multitasking seems to be a habit shared by many, but scientific studies have suggested that this can be counterproductive. It might make you feel productive, but it's not necessarily something that the brain is able to do well. Two different thoughts aren't able to run continuously at the same time with a high level of success. Concentrating on what's in front of you will allow the mind to get to a point of higher-level thinking to utilise your creativity. This is especially important during a creative slump. If everything seems to be working against you, it can help to focus on one task.

Make a list of all the tasks ahead of you, creative or otherwise. Don't think about the order at this stage, just get everything down and out of your head

....

....

....

....

....

....

Make a second list, putting the items in order of priority. If there are tasks that will distract you from free thinking if you don't attend to them, then put these at the top and schedule time to do them first. Reassure yourself that there's time for all the things on your list, it's okay to spend some time creatively

....

....

....

....

....

....

3. Make a plan or throw it away
Concentration can help you push through difficult moments, but it can be hard to figure out what to focus on. If you're struggling to keep your mind on your task, try the following tips:

- Set a strict schedule for your creative output for a day or two and stick to it, no matter what.

- Try some proven methods – the Pomodoro Technique, for example, uses a cooking timer to break down work into short intervals. Or try a productivity app that helps to structure your day. These can help keep you in the mindset needed to think deeply about a subject.

- Try throwing the schedule out of the window. Let any feelings guide you and explore random thoughts. They may seem silly, but that could lead to a surprising innovation or a shift in perspective.

- Accept your feelings – creative slumps can create feelings of hopelessness, but viewing them as natural or as a challenge to expand creative thinking flips the situation and maintains a healthy working pattern.

- Don't despair – keep in mind how good you'll feel once you get back into the flow and keep going.

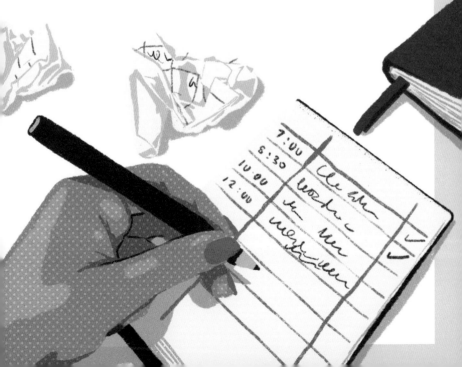

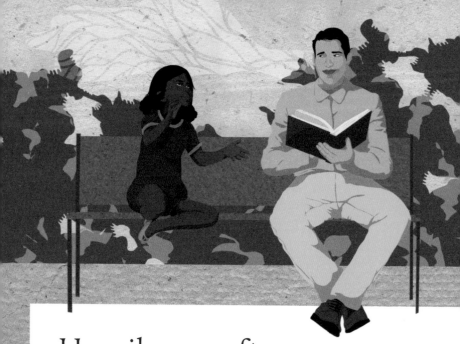

Happily ever after

People have told stories for millions of years and written them for thousands, using them to make sense of the world. At their best they can spark ideas, unite people and bring meaning and fulfilment

The anecdote your family regales around the dinner table. The fairytale you tell your children before bed. The self-image you hold in your head. The political speech wheeled out before an election. The front page of the newspaper. The latest must-watch television series. A new advertising campaign. What do they all have in common? Storytelling. The medium may change, but the power of stories is universal.

A vehicle for understanding

Anthropologists say that storytelling is central to human existence and has been a part of society since the Stone Age. People use stories to make sense of the world and to share that understanding with others, in the process connecting to a larger self and universal truths. From early creation stories and religious parables to modern fables, stories are a means of understanding. 'Creating stories about sea creatures, mythical gods or animals real and imagined, is a lighter way of expressing our own pains, worries and moral dilemmas,' says Barbara Bloomfield from Lapidus, a writing-for-wellbeing organisation. Stories help you to navigate some of those worries in a form that feels more palatable.

Shared experience

Stories provide a space in which to explore the interconnectedness of things, and through that experience, you learn. As the late American poet Stanley Kunitz wrote in *The Layers*: 'I have walked through many lives, some of them my own, and I am not who I was.'

George Murphy is a writer, storyteller and chairman of Shaggy Dog Storytellers, a group promoting oral storytelling in West Yorkshire. He used to tell an ancient Italian story, called *The Land Where No One Ever Dies*, to older primary school pupils. 'Of course, death always wins in the end,' he says. 'But the story provided an opportunity for children to confront their own fears and share their experiences of the demise of much-loved pets and the even more painful loss of family members. An ancient tale enabled them to address an issue that is too often hidden away.'

Having the right story to turn to in times of need can make coping with difficult times easier. Make a note of some of the tales that have brought you comfort and create a therapeutic library that you can turn to whenever you're in need

....

....

....

....

....

....

....

....

....

....

Making connections

As well as the personal benefits, stories offer opportunities for groups and society to come together. It's no coincidence that the stories in the Old Testament led to the ancient Hebrews acting as a unified society devoted to God and his commandments. Similarly, the stories of King Arthur and St George have become rooted in a collective identity of Britain.

Glenys Newton is a member of Cambridge Storytellers: 'By sharing our stories we forge friendships, families and communities. We learn about the lives and the culture of others and a communion is formed,' she says. Key to the society's work and events is the oral tradition, and the interaction between the speaker and the listener. It's in the process of telling that connection takes place. Sharing tales allows people to pool ideas and thoughts, and build dialogue. Societies, and groups within them, are built on shared narratives.

Chemical reaction

According to research by psychologist Dan Johnson, published in the journal *Basic and Applied Social Psychology*, reading fiction increases empathy with others and outsiders. He and his team studied the MRI scans of individuals and found that the parts of the brain related to connection, relationships and empathy were activated when they were exposed to stories.

Studies have also shown that the same hormonal changes occur when hearing or reading a story as would be seen if the event was taking place in real life:

- Cortisol – is produced when something warrants your attention – for example, distress.
- Oxytocin – allows you to feel empathy with a character and promotes pro-social behaviour.
- Dopamine – is released when you are rewarded by emotionally charged events.

Stories can make you kinder and, in turn, improve the society in which you live.

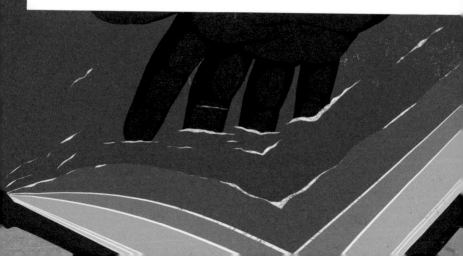

PROVIDING STRUCTURE

One way in which stories help promote happiness is through the sense of order they provide. With their beginning, middle, end and (mostly) resolution, there's a certain sense of comfort that arises from their predictable nature. You can experience difficult situations or emotions within their safety net, confident in the knowledge that all will be sorted by the end.

    Choose an episode from your own life and distil it down into three paragraphs, a beginning, a middle and an ending. It can help to start by choosing a contained but formative experience, like a first day at school or college, or the day you passed your driving test, moved house or climbed a mountain.

Beginning

....

....

....

....

Middle

....

....

....

....

Ending

....

....

....

....

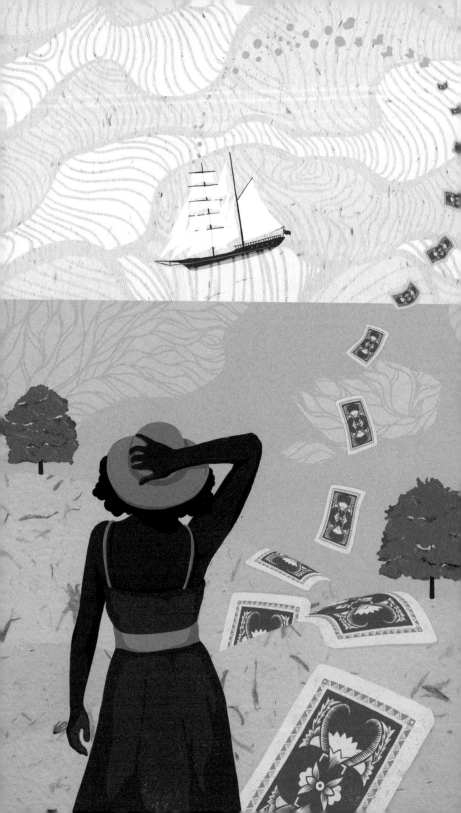

A PATH TO WELLBEING

As a means of bringing people together, a way to discover new ideas or to make sense of the world, a source of inspiration or an opportunity for exploration, stories are hard to beat. Philip Pullman, author of fantasy trilogy *His Dark Materials*, once said: 'After nourishment, shelter and companionship, stories are the thing we need most in the world.' Stories have been wielding their power for thousands of years and their impact remains potent, maybe it's time to tell yours.

My story

....

....

....

....

....

....

....

....

....

....

....

....

....

....

Smell your way to happiness

Whether it's looking at photos, listening to evocative music or snuggling up to the warmth and softness of a pet, our senses constantly gratify us. But what about our sense of smell? Is it just an incidental function that supports all the others or could the olfactory receptors be the route to contentment?

Guess how many different aromas are recognisable? Scientists previously thought that the human nose could detect about 10,000 different smells. But 2014 research from the Rockefeller University in New York revealed that humans can, in fact, smell at least one trillion distinct scents. In addition, other studies have shown that people remember smells with 65 per cent accuracy after a year compared with visual recall, which is about 50 per cent after three months. Smell, it seems, reigns supreme.

The oldest sense

The sense of smell is there for a whole host of reasons, from warning about hazards to enabling the taste and enjoyment of food. As one of the chemical senses – the other being taste – it's used continuously to evaluate the environment for information as well as to indicate things such as the presence of food or another person. In their 1988 paper, *Affect and Memory: Effects of Pleasant and Unpleasant Odors on Retrieval of Happy and Unhappy Memories*, Howard Ehrlichman and Jack N Halpern explain how we can do this without even thinking. It all starts in the womb with the growing foetus learning about odour when flavour compounds from the mother's diet are ingested via the amniotic fluid.

The olfactory system is a fantastic early-warning device but research increasingly shows that it's way more important than just that – it can make you happier and kinder, too. Helen Hopkins, The Balance Coach, says: 'Scent can be essential for triggering happy memories. When we breathe in, the scent goes right to the emotional centre of the brain.'

What does happiness smell like?

Evidence points towards certain smells making people happier, but it also suggests that personal aromas can indicate our own levels of happiness to others. Scientists at Utrecht University in the Netherlands have found that through a process of chemosignalling, people can become 'emotionally synchronised' without even realising it. Researchers collected the sweat of participants in different states – happy, fearful and neutral – by placing pads under their armpits while they watched different movie clips.

The pads were then cut up, put into jars and presented to a group of receivers to sniff randomly. While they did this, the researchers measured differences in their facial muscle activity, which was taken as expressing the emotion being experienced, and discovered that exposure to the 'happy' sweat elicited a happier facial expression from the fearful or neutral situations. The researchers said the study, which was published in the journal *Psychological Science*, showed that 'a positive state (happiness) can be transferred by means of odours'.

All in all, being able to smell makes people happier. Helen says: 'Smell really is unique. The slightest whiff of something familiar and we can be carried right back to a person, place or situation, and as though we're actually living through a memory or emotion all over again. I believe it can promote greater happiness and uplift the spirits.'

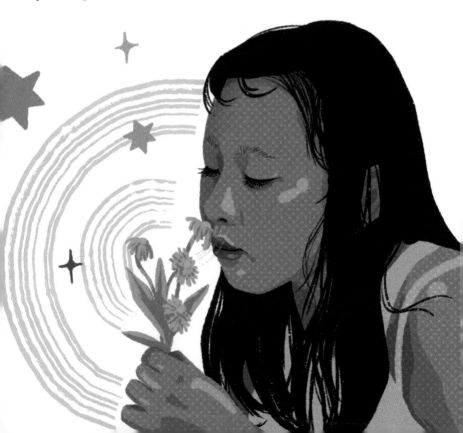

SCENTS PROVEN BY SCIENCE

A range of studies has found that smells can have a direct impact on mood and hormone production.

- **Lavender** –numerous studies have confirmed that exposure to this herb's smell reduces stress (including in newborn babies).

- **Coffee** – researchers in South Korea discovered that after smelling roasted coffee beans, the stress levels of lab rats decreased.

- **Peppermint** – a study at Wheeling University in the US found that the smell of peppermint boosts mood and motivation in competitive athletes.

- **Baking bread** – the University of Southern Brittany found that the smell of baking bread made people kinder to strangers. When eight volunteers stood outside a bakery and dropped a personal item on the floor, 77 per cent of strangers helped them recover their lost items. This is contrasted with just 52 per cent when the volunteers were outside a clothes shop.

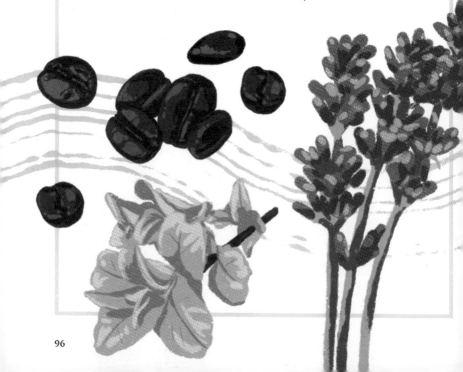

FOUR OLFACTORY WONDERS TO BOOST WELLBEING

- **Fall asleep to sweet fragrances.** A German study showed that smell could influence the quality of dreams. Volunteers had the smell of roses or rotten eggs wafted in front of their noses during their REM (dreaming) sleep. Scientists discovered that the emotional tone of their dreams was more positive with the flowers. Put a vase of fragrant flowers or a scented candle next to your bed before you go to sleep at night for a pleasant slumber.

- **Change your sheets.** Research by Bupa in 2015 found that 'sleeping in a freshly made bed' was right at the top of the list of 50 things that make people happy. So as well as putting flowers in your room, change your bedding regularly to help make you happier.

- **Have a happy kitchen.** The smell of freshly baked bread, bacon sandwiches and fine wine made people happy, according to the Bupa research. A 2014 study at the University of London's Centre for the Study of the Senses discovered that the 'happiest fruit' is the strawberry – 86 per cent of people felt more relaxed by simply thinking about eating one. Researcher Professor Barry Smith said it's the distinctive strawberry smell that evoked happy memories. But think about where you're eating your happy-smelling foods – the study found the sounds of a picnic and lawnmower made strawberries taste fruitier than when people listened to office and commuting noises.

- **Create your own smell library.** Studies demonstrate that a massive 75 per cent of emotions are triggered by smell. For example, research has shown that one of the most evocative smells from childhood is crayons – 85 per cent of people remembered their childhood when they caught the waft of them. It could be that crayons are a positive trigger for you, but it might equally be Tarmac or freshly cut grass.

USE SCENTS TO ANCHOR YOUR FEELINGS OF JOY

Psychotherapist Nick Davies says: 'You can use a neurolinguistic programming technique called anchoring to recreate positive moods.' Here's how to use your sense of smell to reconnect to uplifting emotions.

- Choose a scent that you enjoy, ideally pick one that doesn't already have a specific memory or emotion attached to it. Have your scent of choice ready, but keep a lid on it or put it at a distance so you can't yet smell it.

- Recall a time when you experienced a positive emotional state, ideally one that you would like to be able to recreate at will. Write down everything you saw, heard and felt at the time.

....

....

....

....

....

....

....

....

....

....

....

....

....

- Indicate the level of your emotional state on a scale of 0 to 10 – with 0 being no feeling at all and 10 being the best you've ever felt.

....

- Make the recollection as clear as possible in your mind. The pictures and sounds of your memory should be vibrant and crisp. Allow those great feelings to wash over you again. Before you move on, make sure the experience rates as at least seven on your positivity scale.

- Sniff the scent deeply as your positive feelings rise to create an association between them.

- Distract yourself by thinking about a random question such as 'What did I have for breakfast?' or 'What was I doing last Tuesday morning?'

- Now, test the anchor by smelling the scent again to see if it connects you to the positive feelings of your previous experience.

- If the connection is not strong enough, repeat the exercise from stage 2 until you can generate the desired emotional state just by sniffing your chosen scent.

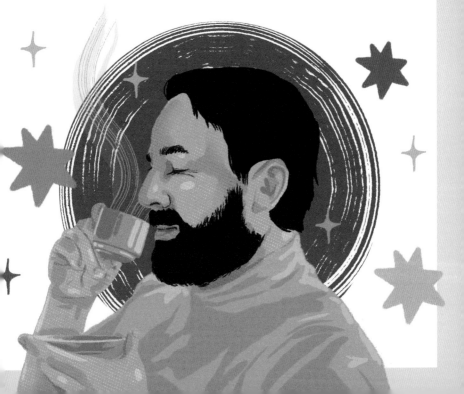

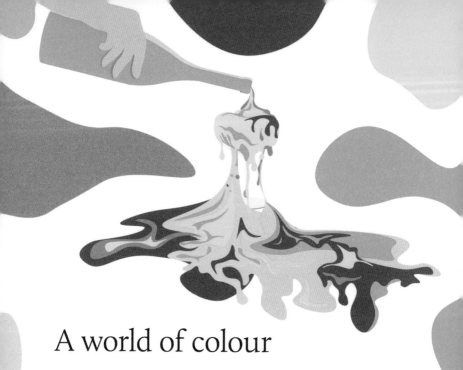

A world of colour

Feeling blue? Seeing red? Green with envy? Colour imbues and surrounds life – and for chromotherapists, it's the perfect tool to ensure you're always in the pink

Yellow peril, purple prose, green-eyed monsters and silver linings – the whole colour spectrum has been entwined with the human condition for thousands of years, whether to denote a psychological state or a physical one. For some, colour is just a mood agent for clever interior design or marketing (orange for optimism, blue for trust). For those who believe in chromotherapy, however, it's a useful tool to restore health and maintain wellbeing.

Much of the modern understanding about colour is a result of one man sticking a needle in his eye. In 1666, Isaac Newton was engaged in a study of the composition of light and optics. In his pamphlet, *Of Colours*, he was trying to establish the properties of colours and whether they originated from within the eye or outside it. His breakthrough moment came when he managed to get sunshine to pass through a prism in a darkened room and it diffracted into the colours of the rainbow. Until that point, it was believed that light was a singular thing, with colours originating from elsewhere in the natural world. The experiments demonstrated that light was a compound of many primary colours, which could be separated or mixed together to form additional hues.

While Newton was interested in the science of colour, ancient civilisations had believed that, physically at least, it was the key to health, happiness and longevity.

Health and hue

In 980AD, the Persian philosopher and physician Avicenna began to catalogue what he determined as the healing properties of individual colours, codifying what would become known as chromotherapy – or using colour to treat illness. In *The Canon of Medicine*, Avicenna developed a chart that showed what he believed was the relationship between colour and the physical condition of the body. He believed red, for instance, could move the blood, while blue or white cooled it and yellow could reduce muscular pain and inflammation.

Meanwhile, Indian physicians who practised Ayurvedic medicine associated individual colours with each of the seven chakras that correspond to specific areas of the body. According to these doctrines, if a chakra is imbalanced or diseased, the application of the appropriate colour can cure or rebalance the chakra and restore health.

COLOUR AND CULTURE

People respond to colour in particular and entrenched ways. This is usually a mix of personal preference, experience, upbringing and cultural differences. Here are some examples of the different ways colours are seen in different parts of the world

- In ancient Egypt, turquoise symbolised fertility.

- In Indonesia, the colour green is forbidden.

- In the Middle East, green represents fertility, luck, wealth and is considered the traditional colour of Islam.

- In China, a man would never wear a green hat because it would signify that he is a cuckold.

- In the west, red is the colour of passion, love and danger, while blue, indigo, grey and silver are seen as tranquil and calming.

- In Asian countries, red stands for good luck, joy and happiness. Asian brides often wear red on their wedding day.

SHADES OF MEANING

It can be useful to consider your own immediate associations with each colour and what they represent to you. These might be moods or cultural symbols, such as danger or luck. Make a note of them here

Red ....

....

Orange ....

....

Yellow ....

....

Green ....

....

Blue ....

....

Indigo/Purple ....

....

Violet/Pink ....

....

'Colour is a power which directly influences the soul'

Wassily Kandinsky

FEEL THE RAINBOW

Chromotherapists share much in common with the Ayurvedics in that they believe the human body is receptive to colour, which is part of the electromagnetic spectrum, as a form of energy. The theory behind chromotherapy lies in the fact that all matter – cells, organs, tissues and atoms – is composed of energy. Bodies that suffer imbalance or illness in a particular area or organ can be retuned with a dose of a corresponding colour that is administered in the form of coloured light or crystal.

Everyone responds to colour differently. To use colour to enhance happiness, experiment by looking, with a relaxed gaze, at a range of different colours and shades. Try to set aside the associations you've listed above, and just sit with the colours for two or three minutes. Write down the feelings each colour evokes

Shades of red ....

....

Shades of orange and gold ....

....

Shades of yellow ....

....

Shades of green ....

....

Shades of blue ....

....

Shades of purple ....

....

Shades of pink ....

....

'And forget not that the earth delights to feel your bare feet and the winds long to play with your hair'

Khalil Gibran

Sole to soul

How going barefoot and walking mindfully can be just the right therapy for your feet – and your whole body

The feet are one of the most nerve-packed parts of the body, so it's little wonder they're so sensitive. Each foot contains a set of strong ligaments, muscles and tendons as well as a whopping 26 bones. In fact, the feet and hands account for more than half the bones in the human body.

Recent Harvard research reveals that people who are habitually barefoot walk in a very different way to those who wear shoes, reducing the overall amount of force through the body as each foot meets the ground. This can improve a person's gait and means there's a smaller risk of muscular problems as a result of better biomechanics.

Although humans evolved without footwear, nowadays, the majority of us have our feet well covered with socks and shoes for most of our waking hours. As a result, we have become disconnected from our natural environment. Our feet are the gateway to proprioception – our awareness of where our body is in relation to our surroundings – so it's little wonder that we can sometimes feel ungrounded.

Joanne [Joe] Bull, a York-based massage therapist and yoga teacher is a great believer in the power of the feet to give your overall wellbeing a boost: 'I spend the majority of my day barefoot and have noticed a significant difference in my body and mind when I have to wear shoes and socks. I feel less "present", my body less open and my feet feel compressed, even in the roomiest of footwear,' she says.

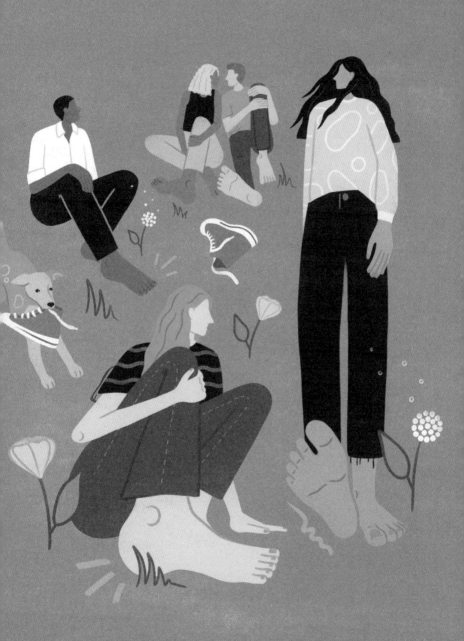

Point of connection

'Grounding' or 'earthing', as it has become known, basically means allowing the skin to be in direct contact with the earth, enabling you to connect with your surroundings in a more mindful way. Research cited by the *Journal of Environmental and Public Health* claims that going barefoot enables you to draw electrons from the earth, which change the electrical activity in your brain, providing an improved sense of wellbeing, as well as physiological changes such as boosting red blood cells and enabling better sleep.

But if drawing energy from the earth sounds far-fetched, there's still a lot to be said for taking a barefoot walk. Remember childhood summer holidays when days were spent playing outdoors, without shoes? Springy daisy-filled grass or soft damp sand beneath your toes and the smell of warm earth elicited a wonderful sense of relaxation and freedom.

Think back to these barefoot experiences and make a list of your five favourite sole sensations so that you can look out for opportunities to recreate them

➤ ....

....

➤ ....

....

➤ ....

....

➤ ....

....

➤ ....

....

➤ ....

....

➤ ....

....

THINK ON YOUR FEET

- Start by taking some slow, mindful steps around the room.

- Notice where you feel your weight land in each foot – is it on the ball of your foot or the heel? Can you feel more weight in one foot than the other?

- Notice the sensations in each foot as it makes contact with the ground.

- Experiment with changing the way each foot connects with the ground – for example, shifting weight from the outside to the inside and front to back.

- Experience the sensations that spread across your feet and up your legs.

- Practise pressing each toe in the ground individually.

- Notice how this affects the rest of your body.

- Breathe deeply to connect with your movement.

- Experience a sense of grounding calm and enjoy.

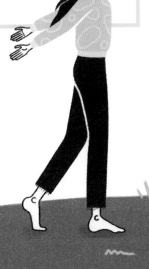

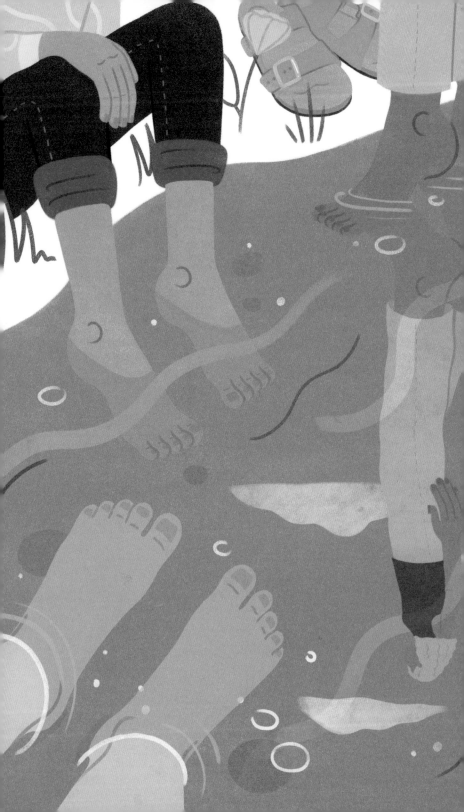

TOUCH YOUR TOES

Another way to get in touch with your feet is with a foot massage. The simple act of touching your own feet can be deeply relaxing. Sit in a position where you're comfortably supported, crossing one foot over the opposite knee or in front of your body, and give this a try

- Use both hands to cup one foot.

- Use both thumbs to gently press into the heels with a slow, rhythmic motion.

- Slowly move the thumbs down towards the arch of the foot, move from the inside to the outside of the foot, continuing to press gently.

- Move down to the soft, sensitive area beneath the ball of the foot, gently continuing the padding action with the thumbs.

- Notice a releasing sensation in each area as you move down the foot.

- Gently press the thumbs into the ball of the foot with a soft, circular motion.

- Use both thumbs and first fingers to massage each toe in turn.

- Carefully thread the fingers between the toes and move the toes with a gentle back-and-forth fanning action.

- Finish by gently patting the sole and top of the foot using both hands.

- Breathe deeply and take a few minutes to absorb the sensations and feelings of relaxation. Repeat with the other foot.

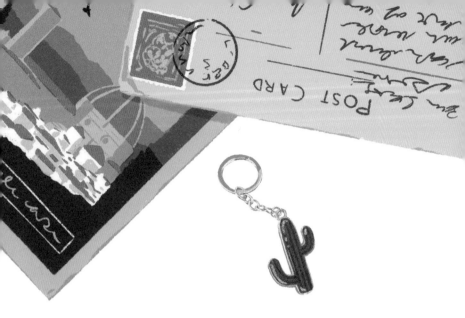

Connecting to collecting

The joyful art of building, organising and curating a collection

Are you a falerist or a plangonologist? Do you consider yourself to be a
deltiologist in the making? It may be that you are and just didn't know it, as
they're all fairly obscure terms to describe people who collect particular objects.
Being a collector, though, is about much more than curious terminology or the
physical act of accumulating stuff. There's a strong emotional side to it, too.
There's joy to be found in starting a collection and a sense of achievement in
building it up; organising and arranging it can be comforting and provide a
sense of wellbeing. Then there's the satisfaction of displaying a collection in
a beautiful or unexpected way.

The personal touch
Collections are often about personal connections. It may be a reminder of
a happy, important or comforting time in life – the books read when growing
up, action figures played with in earlier years or a coin collection that was
kick-started by a relative. Keeping those items close, looking at them and
holding them can bring back special memories.

It may be that a collection is borne out of an attraction to the way something
looks, such as the design of certain perfume bottles or the intricate patterns on
decorative plates. There are items that have a particular draw because of what
they represent – military medals are testament to tales of heroism, bravery and
certain moments in history, while special-edition stamps mark the notable
achievements of significant people around the world.

BECOME A CURATOR

Make a list of five items that are precious to you and the good feelings
or happy times that you associate with them. They might be one-offs
at the moment, but they could be the first piece in your collection

▶ ....
....
....

▶ ....
....
....

▶ ....
....
....

▶ ....
....
....

▶ ....
....
....

Interaction and discovery

The joy of collecting can extend beyond a connection to certain items. It can be a great way to connect with other people, too. Antique and vintage fairs, car boot sales, flea markets and specialist shops provide more than just an opportunity to find an object, they're also a chance to chat with like-minded collectors. Sharing photos of your pieces on social media and discussing them on dedicated forums can extend your network and lead to new friendships. Having a collection on display at home, and adding new items to it, is also a great point of discussion for visiting friends and family.

Building a collection can be a wonderful tool for learning and discovery – it's an opportunity to uncover everything from how the items you've acquired were made to the history of who made them.

Find out as much as you can about three of the items on your list on the previous page. If you don't know the details, the internet can be a great resource

Item 1

Name ....

....

Date made ....

Place of origin ....

Any other details ....

....

....

....

....

Item 2

Name ....

....

Date made ....

Place of origin ....

Any other details ....

....

....

....

....

Item 3

Name ....

....

Date made ....

Place of origin ....

Any other details ....

....

....

....

....

....

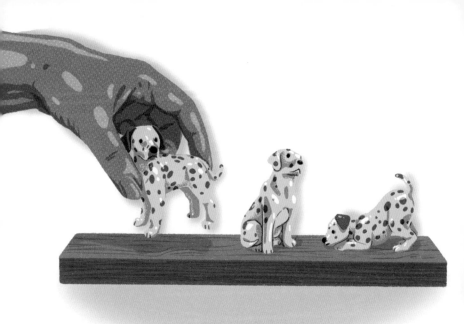

Visual appeal

One of the most enjoyable aspects of building a collection can be contemplating how best to arrange and display it. The act of organising it can be richly rewarding, providing a sense of order and focus.

In this digital age, perhaps there is even greater comfort to be found in the physicality of a collection. There are times when holding or rearranging the objects can have a calming, almost therapeutic effect. Plus, ordering and displaying them in a particular way can be visually pleasing – you can group everyday objects in such a way that they become a thing of beauty.

Putting the items on display in a particular way – on a shelving unit, in a curio cabinet, hung on a wall, stacked on a table – can add to the collection's aesthetic appeal or mean that it is viewed from a new and different perspective.

It may be that your collection is edited for display and you choose to put out only one section of it – the items that mean the most or that look nicest together. It could be that you rotate your display, having certain items out at particular times, then swapping them. The guiding principle should be that the way you arrange it should bring a sense of satisfaction and contentment.

A sense of self

A collection can be so much more than a grouping of objects – it can be a physical representation of your interests, your personality, your identity. It can anchor you to an important time or person in your life. Building it can give you a sense of achievement and sharing it with others is often rewarding. If you already have a collection, you might want to find a fresh, new way of displaying it. If you've yet to start one, give it some thought, consider the items to which you're emotionally drawn and look at the objects already around you – perhaps you've begun your collection without even realising it.

10 CURIOUS TERMS FOR COLLECTORS

- Copoclephile: keyrings

- Deltiologist: postcards

- Digitabulist: thimbles

- Falerist: medals, badges and pins

- Helixophile: corkscrews

- Notaphilist: banknotes

- Pannapictagraphist: comics

- Phillumenist: matchboxes

- Plangonologist: dolls

- Vexillophile: flags

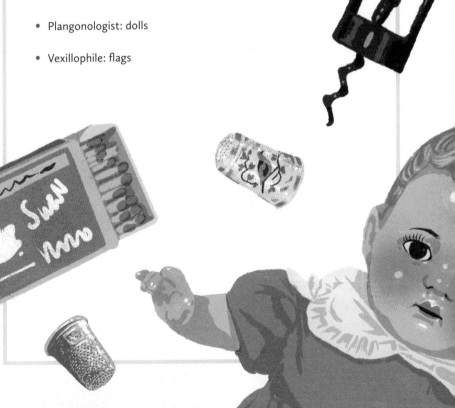

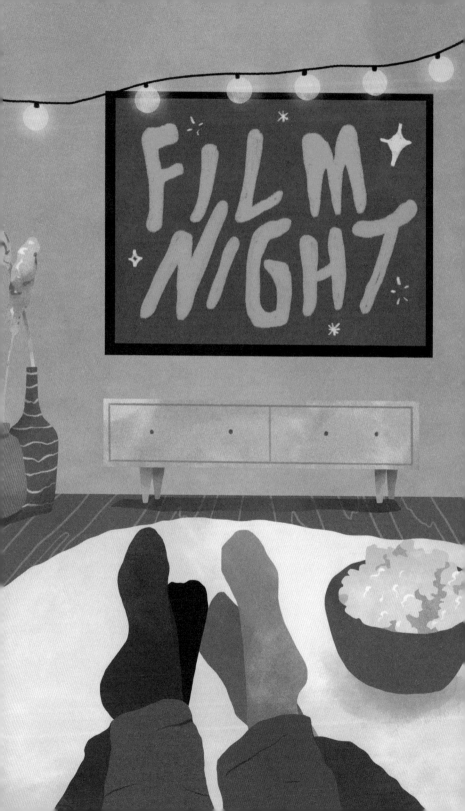

'Every great film should seem new every time you see it'

Roger Ebert

Great escapes

A film can transport you to a different world or make you look anew at your own. It can lift your spirits, shift your perspective and make you laugh

The very act of watching a film can be richly rewarding – setting aside time to watch one can be an indulgent treat if alone and a unifying experience if with others. Comedy, of course, can provide an instant bounce. But recent research has found that even emotional wringers can trigger the release of feel-good, pain-numbing endorphins in the brain.

An Oxford University study, published in the journal *Royal Society Open Science* in 2016, found that watching sad films together can boost feelings of group bonding and increase pain tolerance. It's thought that film-watching could provide long-term therapeutic benefits too, with proponents of cinema therapy using films as an aid to counselling and as a means of identifying certain feelings or behaviours.

A connection to a particular film, and its ability to transport the viewer or evoke an emotion, can be immediate but lasting and profound. As Oscar-winning film-maker Martin Scorsese has shared: 'Movies touch our hearts, awaken our vision, and change the way we see things. They take us to other places. They open doors and minds. Movies are the memories of our lifetime. We need to keep them alive.'

Here are 10 exceptional films that have the power to uplift, present a message of mindfulness or simply provide an opportunity to escape. Sit back, relax and press play...

Groundhog Day (1993)

Arrogant Pittsburgh weatherman Phil Connors (Bill Murray) is sent to a small Pennsylvania town to cover the Groundhog Day festival, where he scorns the locals and his new producer Rita (Andie MacDowell). When a blizzard forces him to stay in the town another night, however, he finds he's trapped in a 24-hour loop, waking up on Groundhog Day morning over and over again. At first, he takes his daily reboot as an opportunity to live without consequence or remorse, but the repetition eventually breaks him down and his sharp edges are softened. Murray shines in a film that's generous with humour and warm-heartedness – his character stops looking for reasons to be unhappy tomorrow and starts finding reasons to be happy today.

Big Fish (2003)

Edward Bloom has spent a lifetime telling tall tales about his adventurous younger years, but his son, Will, has tired of the far-fetched stories and the pair have become estranged. When they're brought back together, Will has only a few days to mend their relationship and learn whether there's any substance to his dad's flights of fancy, recounted in a series of lively flashbacks. Master of the fantastical, Tim Burton's film is full of magical moments and colourful characters, but its breezy soundtrack and whimsical wanderings are underpinned by lofty themes – destiny, loss, love and truth among them. The threads of Edward's stories are woven together wonderfully in the film's touching final scenes.

Amélie (2001)

Jean-Pierre Jeunet's romantic comedy follows Parisian waitress Amélie Poulain, who, having led an isolated life as a child, feels compelled to improve the lives of those around her – from a lovelorn colleague to an embittered neighbour. For Amélie (played with wide-eyed wonderment by Audrey Tautou), there's interest and intrigue around every corner, marvel and magic in the mundane – she finds pure joy in the crunch of a crème brûlée under a spoon. When Amélie helps a blind man along the street, she describes to him in glorious detail all that surrounds him. Hers is a world of colour, noise and texture – she opens her eyes, and eventually her heart, to a life that presents an opportunity for adventure at every turn.

Local Hero (1983)

Eccentric Texan oil tycoon Felix Happer sets his sights on buying up the small Scottish fishing village of Ferness to establish a new refinery. He sends one of his US executives, 'Mac' MacIntyre, to convince the locals to sell up and move away. Bill Forsyth's drama follows Mac as he 'goes native', teaming up with Scottish oil rep Oldsen and setting out to get the people of Ferness to sign on the dotted line. As the days go by, Mac finds himself increasingly drawn to the villagers and the beauty of the place. Forsyth's script is subtle, smart and funny, and there is a lyrical quality to the film's gentle pace. Time spent with the people of Ferness is time well spent indeed.

Some Like It Hot (1959)

Chicago musicians Joe (Tony Curtis) and Jerry (Jack Lemmon) are rumbled as they witness a gangster mob exacting revenge on their rivals. The pair need to get out of town quick, so don wigs and dresses and present themselves as Josephine and Daphne in order to join an all-female musical group heading to Florida. At their Miami hotel, Joe tries to woo ukulele player and singer Sugar Kane (Marilyn Monroe) by adopting the additional identity of oil heir Junior, while Jerry finds that his Daphne has drawn the amorous attention of wealthy older man Osgood. It's impossible not to get carried along by the verve of Billy Wilder's rollicking comedy classic, which is rightly remembered for, among many fabulously farcical moments, its final line: 'Well, nobody's perfect.'

Cinema Paradiso (1988)

Film-maker Salvatore Di Vita has been estranged from the people of his Sicilian village hometown for 30 years. When his mother reaches out to him with news of the passing of an old friend, he recalls, in flashbacks, his own formative years. As a six-year-old, spirited Salvatore (nicknamed Toto) is besotted with film and the village cinema – a lively place where locals of all ages come together to laugh, cry and shout at the big screen. Toto gets under the feet of projectionist Alfredo and the pair form an unshakeable bond over the years that follow. Giuseppe Tornatore's Italian drama is a love letter to cinema, touchingly wistful and nostalgic. The film ends, but its heartfelt depiction of film as a force that brings people together lingers long afterwards.

The Princess Bride (1987)

Fairy tales have long captured the imagination with far-off lands and improbable characters. Rob Reiner's fantasy adventure, based on the novel of the same name by William Goldman, does exactly that, with a knowing joviality that's hard to resist. The film opens with a grandpa arriving at the bedside of his poorly grandson to read him a book, *The Princess Bride*, and it's this tale that plays out on screen. The story is a familiar one – a lowly farmhand becomes a dashing hero as he sets about rescuing his one true love from a ragtag band of outlaws and a sinister prince – but the film has an enduring freshness. It's a fantasy that's infinitely quotable and, in the tradition of all good fairy tales, effortlessly enchanting.

Before Sunrise (1995)

Richard Linklater's romantic drama forgoes bells and whistles for the appealingly simple storytelling technique of two people walking and talking. Those two people are early twentysomethings American tourist Jesse (Ethan Hawke) and French student Céline (Julie Delpy) who, by chance, find themselves sitting opposite each other on a train bound for Vienna. Their instant and easy rapport sees them spontaneously agreeing to spend the evening together exploring the city. The pair wander the streets of Vienna, discussing their thoughts, feelings, hopes and dreams as the clock ticks down on their time together. There is a simple, believable charm to this story of two people who live in the moment and form an unexpectedly deep and meaningful connection.

Eddie the Eagle (2016)

In 1973, a young, physically impaired Eddie Edwards puts on his coat and declares that he's heading to Rome to take part in the Olympics. He's soon back at home, but over the years that follow, loses none of his burning desire to become an Olympian. Convinced he can make it as a ski jumper, Eddie decamps to a training facility in Germany, where he convinces a gruff ex-ski jumper to mentor him in the run-up to the 1988 Calgary Winter Olympics. Dexter Fletcher's affectionate biopic follows Eddie (Taron Egerton) as he seeks to conquer not just the slopes but also the derision of the sporting establishment – and, though it grants itself poetic licence in the telling of a true story, it's in capturing Eddie's resilience in the pursuit of his seemingly impossible dream that it soars.

Singin' in the Rain (1952)

It's impossible not to get swept along by the energy and joy that course through MGM's classic musical about Hollywood's transition from silent to sound in the 1920s. Don Lockwood (Gene Kelly) and leading lady Lina Lamont (Jean Hagen) find their futures as box-office draws at risk after the disastrous test screening of their first 'talkie', so studio heads decide to reshoot it as a musical and dub over Lina's shrill voice with that of Don's love interest, Kathy (Debbie Reynolds). *Singin' in the Rain*'s song-and-dance numbers are so rich in comedy and full of bounce that the urge to get up, get out and jump in puddles is almost overwhelming.

WONDERS OF THE BIG SCREEN

Note down some of your favourite films and how they make you feel

On a high

Sometimes, true happiness comes from stepping back to take in the whole, beautiful picture

When Ron Garan set out for work in June 2008, it was never going to be a normal day at the office. The Nasa astronaut was about to clamp himself to the end of a robotic arm that would travel in an arc above the International Space Station (ISS) in a manoeuvre known as the windshield wiper. Close to the peak of this arc, Garan was met with a view of the ISS some 100ft below, and the Earth 240 miles away. 'It was as if time stood still, and I was flooded with emotion and awareness,' he later recalled.

Humans first saw Earth from space in 1946, when a modified movie camera was mounted on a captured Nazi V-2 rocket and launched from a missile range in New Mexico. When the rocket came down minutes later, the camera revealed black-and-white images of the Earth's curvature from 65 miles up. One of the most iconic shots of the planet was taken by the crew of the last Apollo mission (Apollo 17) on its way to the Moon in 1972. Dubbed *The Blue Marble*, it shows the Earth in its entirety, in full colour. Looking at it triggers various responses but most include a new appreciation of the planet's fragile beauty and a profound sense of peace.

A shift in perspective

A few years after *The Blue Marble* was taken, Harvard graduate Frank White was flying in a passenger plane north of Washington DC. Looking out of the window he saw the Capitol and Washington Monument 30,000ft below and suddenly found it absurd that these human ants were making life-changing decisions and taking themselves so seriously. At the same time, he knew that once the plane touched down, this physical overview would vanish and he would return to being one of the ants. The experience led him to suggest that our philosophical view of the world is dependent on our physical perspective.

Further insights came as the plane flew over the western states. At this point, Frank began to liken himself to a time traveller. Looking at the network of roads beneath him, he could see which cars were going to pass each other miles before the drivers could – in a way, he could see into the future: 'From the airplane, the message that scientists, philosophers, spiritual teachers and systems theorists have been trying to tell us for centuries was obvious, everything is interconnected and interrelated.'

Inner space

To support his theory that the physical has a profound effect on the philosophical, Frank spoke to more than 20 astronauts and cosmonauts and recorded their testimonies for his book, *The Overview Effect: Space Exploration and Human Evolution*. Apollo 9 astronaut 'Rusty' Schweickart describes how the borders enforced on land seem meaningless when considered from space. 'When you go around the Earth in an hour and a half, you begin to recognise that your identity is with that whole thing... You look down there and you can't imagine how many borders and boundaries you cross, again and again and again, and you don't even see them.'

Each astronaut has a different way of describing their experiences and their ability to translate this particular encounter into words varies. What makes it harder is that there is nothing on Earth to compare it to. The view of Earth from space is described as 'overwhelming', 'tremendous' and 'a heart-stopper'. The one thing these space explorers all agree on is that despite the pictures and maps they studied pre-flight, nothing prepared them for the spectacle of seeing Earth from space. What's more, many of them felt changed by it.

Frank calls this change 'the overview effect', something he describes as a 'cognitive shift in awareness' accompanied by feelings of 'awe for the planet, a profound understanding of the interconnection of all life, and a renewed sense of responsibility for taking care of the environment'.

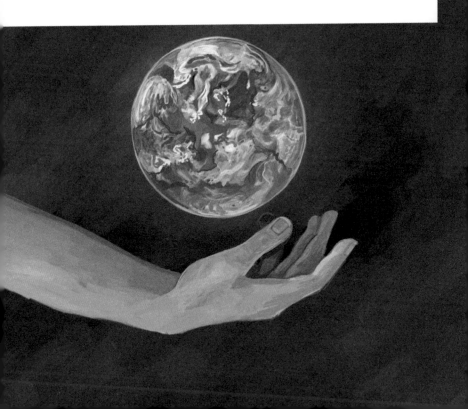

A DIFFERENT VIEW

Think back through your life to a time when you've felt your perspective on life change suddenly. It might have been through seeing the landscape from a new vantage point or through witnessing something that expanded your world view

Ask yourself:

How did I see the world before this experience?

....

....

....

....

....

....

....

What caused the moment of realisation?

....

....

....

....

....

....

....

How did this shift in perspective change me?

....

....

....

....

....

....

....

....

....

....

....

....

....

....

A bird's-eye view

Clearly, you don't need to go into orbit to get a taste of the overview effect. Looking at Nasa's image archive (nasa.gov) or listening to first-hand accounts from astronauts can lead to feelings of awe. One of the best ways to experience interconnectedness is to meditate on the subject. And if you start thinking of the planet as a unified whole rather than fractured parts, you might devise small solutions that could make global improvements. 'Each and every one of us is riding through the universe together on this spaceship we call Earth,' says Ron. 'We are all in this together.' Sometimes we have to step back to see our way forward.

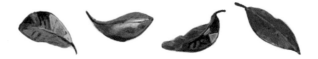

TREE OF LIFE

By focusing on interconnectedness, you are reminded of your relationship to the planet, and everything that draws sustenance and life from it, which can bring a sense of deep contentment. This meditation requires you to find a suitable tree to represent planet Earth, and to sit in front of it for roughly 20 minutes

- Assume a comfortable sitting position. Keep your spine straight and relax your shoulders, letting your shoulder blades roll back and down. Rest your hands where they feel most comfortable. Make any adjustments you need.

- Take five deep breaths, in through the nose and out through the mouth. Keep your eyes open and your gaze soft and steady.

- Bring your attention to the natural rhythm of your breath. Find an area where you can feel it most strongly and rest your awareness there. Pay attention to the full in-breath and the full out-breath. Notice the spaces in between, the gaps at the top of the in-breath and the gaps at the bottom of the out-breath.

- Gaze at the tree in front of you and see it as a complete world, like the Earth. Let your focus be soft. Become aware of all your fields of vision, including your peripheral vision.

- Consider all of the elements that come together to enable this tree to live: the roots that absorb moisture and dissolve minerals from the soil; the trunk that supports the limbs while transporting nutrients from the roots to the leaves; the bark that protects it from external attack; the buds that develop into new leaves. The natural relationships creating a complete ecosystem.

- Now contemplate the sunlight the tree needs to trigger photosynthesis. Think about the rain it requires for moisture and the wind that disperses its seeds. Consider the interdependent nature of these elements.

- Bring to mind the insects and birds that feast on the tree, eating leaves and berries, spreading seeds, guaranteeing its survival. Think of the fungi that utilise the tree, breaking down organic matter and enriching the soil.

- If your attention wavers, notice where it has gone and bring it back to focusing on the tree and interconnectedness. If the mind wanders a thousand times, bring it back a thousand times.

- Now let go of any focus on interconnectedness, and allow the mind to wander wherever it wants to. Stay this way for a few moments.

- Slowly bring your attention to the point of contact between your body and the ground. Move your fingers and toes gently. Come out of the meditation slowly and deliberately.

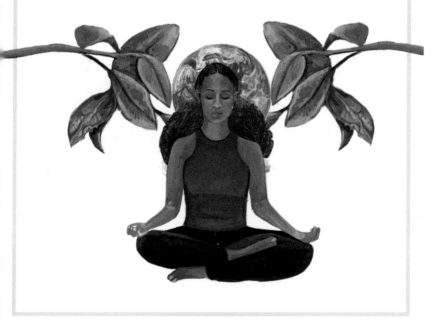

Breathe

BREATHE is a trademark of Guild of Master Craftsman Publications Ltd

First published 2022 by
Ammonite Press
an imprint of Guild of Master Craftsman Publications Ltd
Castle Place, 166 High Street, Lewes, East Sussex BN7 1XU, United Kingdom

www.ammonitepress.com
www.breathemagazine.com

Compiled by Chloe Rhodes
Editorial: Catherine Kielthy, Jane Roe, Josie Fletcher
Words credits: Dean Agius, Jade Angeles Fitton, Francesca Baker, Tracy Calder, Jasmine Harris,
Emma Newlyn, Martha Roberts, Simone Scott, Carol Anne Strange, Julian Venables,
Angela Watt, Janette Wolf

Illustrations: Holly Astle, Katherine Buchanan, Kathrin Lang, Amy Leonard, Steph Mole, Irina Perju,
Silvia Stecher, Kate Styling, Sara Thielker, Michelle Urra, Kimberley Laura Walker
Cover illustration: Maggie Stephenson

ISBN 978 1 78145 467 1

A catalogue record for this book is available from the British Library.

Breathe Magazine
Publisher: Jonathan Grogan
Designer: Jo Chapman

Colour reproduction by GMC Reprographics
Printed and bound in China

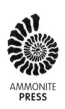

AMMONITE
PRESS